DEPARTMENT OF HEALTH

Changing
Childbirth

Part I: Report of the Expert Maternity Group

≈

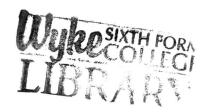

LONDON: The Stationery Office

First published 1993
Sixth impression 2001

ISBN 0 11 321623 8

017834

Contents

Part II: Survey of Good Communications Practice in Maternity Services

(Separately bound)

Message from Virginia Bottomley

I am delighted to see the publication of this refreshing and stimulating review of maternity services. The report gives special attention to the views of women. Pregnancy is not an illness. It is a natural process and the woman should be at the centre of decisions about her care.

At the heart of the NHS reforms is the need for health authorities to listen more and more to what users feel about the health service they require. The thinking in the Group's report is totally in keeping with that philosophy.

The next step is to open up the discussion locally and nationally on the changes needed in maternity services. I want everyone with an interest in these matters – women who use the services, doctors, midwives, health visitors and nurses who deliver them, and NHS managers who purchase and provide them – to debate these changes amongst themselves and let us know how best to proceed.

I am very grateful to Lady Cumberlege and the members of her group for giving us all the opportunity to look to the future in this way. The report will lead to significant improvements in one of the most important aspects of our lives – creating a family.

SECRETARY OF STATE FOR HEALTH

Foreword

Pregnancy is a long and very special journey for a woman. It is a journey of dramatic physical, psychological and social change; of becoming a mother, of redefining family relationships and taking on the long-term responsibility for caring and cherishing a new born child. Generations of women have travelled the same route, but each journey is unique.

Maternity services should support the mother, her baby and her family during this journey with a view to their short-term safety but also their long-term wellbeing. They should help the woman to enjoy pregnancy and childbirth as positive, life-enhancing experiences. No-one has a greater interest in a healthy baby and a happy outcome than the pregnant woman herself, and the Expert Group believes the care should be planned and provided not only around her, but more importantly, in partnership with her.

The care surrounding pregnancy and childbirth takes place in circumstances which distinguish it from almost all other forms of clinical practice. Pregnancy is not a pathological process or a disease. It is a physiological event which occurs in a very high proportion of women during their lifetimes. The majority of pregnancies end normally and without complication.

It may seem paradoxical that, at the time when improved public health and medical knowledge have vastly reduced perinatal and maternal deaths, we should be proposing far-reaching changes to the NHS maternity services. We believe, on the evidence we have seen, that the service could be organised in a way which does not jeopardise safety, yet is kinder, more welcoming and more supportive to the women whose needs it is designed to meet.

The Expert Group is in no doubt that the great majority of clinical care associated with pregnancy and childbirth is carried out by well trained and well qualified professionals who are committed to obtaining the best outcome, as they judge it, for the individuals in their care. However, this clinical care is too often delivered in a way which is determined by a model or pattern of care, more appropriate to states of ill-health than to a physiological process which for the majority results in a normal and uncomplicated outcome.

We are also convinced that there is insufficient scope for women themselves to make truly informed choices. Pregnant women, for the most part, are an informed group, well placed to understand the issues and choices, and to decide for themselves such questions as the type of care they would wish, the sort of professional they would wish to carry it out, the place of delivery, and the degree of intervention.

Considerable evidence examined by the Group points to a set of universal standards that all women want from their maternity care. They want a service that is flexible and responsive to their individual needs, which acknowledges the role of their partners and which communicates effectively. They want improved information that allows them to make informed choices. Above all, women and their partners are seeking a service that is respectful, personalised and kind, which gives them control and makes them feel comfortable in the sense of being at ease in the environment of childbirth and having confidence in their care.

These are simple wants, but in a fragmented service they have proved sadly hard to achieve.

Our report suggests some ways in which these difficulties can be overcome. It acknowledges the good work already being done in all parts of the country upon which the service can build. It recognises that change can only happen if there is a genuine will to achieve it. We believe the will is there. Maternity services are ripe for change in the interests not just of the women they serve, but all those working within the service.

The Expert Group has greatly appreciated the considerable work undertaken efficiently and with good humour by the secretariat at the Department of Health. The team, Jane McKessack, Kate Jackson, John Modle, Joanne Shipton, and Martin Houghton, deserve our heartfelt thanks for their unstinting work.

We would also like to thank all those involved in providing maternity services for making us so welcome during our visits and for going to so much trouble to provide us with objective information on which to judge their work. We are grateful to the many organisations which submitted detailed evidence and briefed us so thoroughly, including all those who contributed to the Consensus Conference.

Julia Cumberlege.

PARLIAMENTARY UNDER SECRETARY OF STATE FOR HEALTH

Expert Maternity Group Membership

Chairman

Baroness Cumberlege, Parliamentary Under Secretary of State for Health

Membership

Mary Anderson, Senior Consultant Obstetrician and Gynaecologist, Lewisham Hospital, London

Simon Court, Consultant Paediatrician, Queen Elizabeth Hospital, Gateshead

Peter Farmer, Management Consultant, Ernst and Young

Eileen Hutton, President, National Childbirth Trust

Liz Lightfoot, Journalist

Lesley Page, Professor of Midwifery, Queen Charlotte's College of Health & Science, Thames Valley University

Kulbir Randhawa, Co-ordinator/Counsellor, Asian Family Counselling Service

Pat Troop, Chief Executive, Cambridge Health Authority and Cambridgeshire FHSA

Gavin Young, General Practitioner, Temple Sowerby, Penrith, Cumbria

Secretariat (Department of Health)

Jane McKessack, Secretary to the Expert Maternity Group

Kate Jackson, Midwifery Development Consultant, Nursing Officer

John Modle, Senior Medical Officer

Joanne Shipton

Martin Houghton

Introduction

1. Enormous improvements have been made in the safety record of maternity services in this country over the last 70 years. Better public health, medical advances and the skill and commitment of all those working within the National Health Service have greatly reduced the number of women who lose their babies. Records show that in 1960 in England and Wales, 30 babies in every 1,000 (total births) were stillborn, or died within the first week. Last year, however, this figure had fallen to fewer than eight in every thousand births. The feelings of grief and distress for mothers and their partners at the death of their babies cannot be over-estimated and it is important that the service strives to bring the rate down still further.

2. Most births – almost 99% – take place in a maternity unit. Current guidance from the Department of Health through the Maternity Services Advisory Committee's 1984 report is that births should take place in hospital. Its report "Maternity Care in Action"[1] gives the following guidance to health authorities: *"As unforeseen complications can occur in any birth, every mother should be encouraged to have her baby in a maternity unit where emergency facilities are available."*

3. In March 1992 the House of Commons Health Select Committee mounted a vigorous challenge to this assumption. In its report "Maternity Services",[2] the Committee stated: *"On the basis of what we have heard, this committee must draw the conclusion that the policy of encouraging all women to give birth in hospitals cannot be justified on grounds of safety."*

4. The Select Committee concluded that a "medical model of care" should no longer drive the service and that women should be given unbiased information and an opportunity for choice in the type of maternity care they receive, including the option, previously largely denied to them, of having their babies at home, or in small maternity units.

5. The Government announced, in its response to the Select Committee's report,[3] that it would set up an expert committee: *"to review policy on NHS maternity care, particularly during childbirth, and to make recommendations."*

---

[1]*Maternity Care in Action,* the report of the Maternity Services Advisory Committee, was produced in three parts:

        Part I - Antenatal Care (1982)
        Part II - Care During Childbirth (1984)
        Part III - Care of Mother and Baby (1985)

[2]Health Committee Second Report, Session 1991-92: Maternity services. HMSO 1992.

[3]Maternity Services: Government Response to the Second Report from the Health Committee, Session 1991-92; Cmnd 2018. HMSO 1992.

6. The Expert Maternity Group was established in October 1992 under the chairmanship of Lady Cumberlege, Parliamentary Under Secretary of State for Health, and drew membership from the women who use NHS maternity services and from those professionals who provide them.

7. The Group recognised that, because of its remit, it would be unable to address issues such as nutrition and socio-economic factors which can influence the outcome of pregnancy and childbirth. We acknowledged that the Government's "Health of the Nation" strategy[4] also highlighted areas of particular relevance to maternity care, such as family planning and the need to reduce smoking and drug abuse which were also beyond our remit.

8. Appropriately, the Group completed its work in nine months. We gathered information and evidence from a wide range of organisations, professional groups and individuals with an interest in maternity care. As well as oral presentations from women using the service, anaesthetists, general practitioners, midwives, obstetricians, paediatricians and other health professionals, we received written evidence from a number of professional and voluntary organisations.[5]

9. Visits to consultant maternity units within general hospitals, small maternity units and midwifery schemes were an integral part of gathering evidence[6]. We were impressed at the level of commitment amongst health professionals and their willingness to discuss improvements to the service, some of which are already under way.

10. In order to explore the relevant issues more fully, a consensus conference was organised by the King's Fund Centre on behalf of the Department of Health. The conference was held on 4 and 5 March 1993 and was attended by more than 400 people. The conference panel produced a consensus statement[7] and this proved extremely valuable in the way it clarified issues and highlighted concerns.

11. To obtain the views of women who are not linked to any particular group or organisation, the Group commissioned a research study by MORI Health Research of mothers who had given birth in England since April 1989. A further survey of Asian and Afro-Caribbean mothers was then

---

[4] *The Health of the Nation: A Strategy for Health in England.* Department of Health 1992.

[5] See Annex 2 for a list of the organisations, representatives of organisations and individuals who gave written and oral evidence to the Group.

[6] See Annex 3 for a list of locations visited by the Group

[7] The consensus statement is reproduced at Annex 4

conducted by MORI to provide specific information about their perceptions of maternity services. Care was taken to interview women in the language with which they felt most familiar.

12.   We considered communication to be of the utmost importance and commissioned SWT Communications to carry out a study. This identified the principles essential for effective communication and in addition identified examples of good practice. The survey is published with this report as we hope it will inspire and encourage others to learn from those who have experienced success in this field.

13.   The Group has already seen the considerable effort that both the purchasers and providers of maternity care have made to respond to the needs and wishes of women but, nevertheless, there is still much that can be done further to improve NHS maternity care.

14.   The Chief Executive of the NHS Management Executive has decided to include maternity services in his Priorities and Planning guidance for 1994/5. This requires health authorities to ensure that the maternity services they purchase are reviewed in the light of our recommendations and to consider, by 1 August 1994, a strategy for implementing any necessary changes. The strategy can then be reflected in contracts for 1995/6.

15.   We believe that women and their families should be at the centre of maternity services which should be planned and provided with their interests and those of their babies in mind. The report begins with a description of this key principle and identifies those aspects of good maternity care which support this vision. It highlights areas where changes will need to be made and finally, sets out the Group's view of action which will bring about a woman centred service.

Woman Centred Care

The Expert Maternity Group set out with the clear objective of improving NHS maternity services. We thought it important that this work did not focus simply on the organisation of the service or the needs of the professionals who work in it. So the Group started its work by asking itself what changes it wanted women to see in maternity services in five years time. As members responded to this question a clear picture emerged. We agreed that maternity care must be woman centred, concentrating on meeting the needs of the women for whom the service is intended. This chapter sets out the key components of such a service.

1.1   Every woman has unique needs. In addition to those arising from her medical history these will derive from her particular ethnic, cultural, social and family background. The services provided should recognise the special characteristics of the population they are designed to serve. They should also be attractive and accessible to all women, particularly those who may be least inclined to use them.

1.2   Information about the local maternity services should be readily available within the community. The woman should be able to choose whether her first contact is with a midwife or her general practitioner, and should feel confident that she will receive accurate and unbiased information from the professional she chooses.

1.3   The woman and, if she wishes, her partner, should be encouraged to be closely involved in the planning of her care. It should be clear to her that her views and wishes, including her desire for a safe outcome, are important and respected. Antenatal care should be designed to ensure that the woman is cared for by professionals who are acceptable to her, and who have the appropriate skills and expertise required in her particular circumstances. She should not feel that she has to choose from one profession and exclude all others. Women should be encouraged to use the service fully and to their advantage.

1.4   Every woman should be given the name of an individual midwife who works locally, to whom she can go for advice and help throughout her pregnancy. In many instances this named midwife will also be the lead professional – undertaking the key role in the planning and provision of care.

1.5   In other circumstances, usually when the pregnancy is more complicated, the lead professional will be an obstetrician. If circumstances change, the lead professional may need to be redesignated. The woman should always be involved when such decisions are to be made. She should feel confident that the professionals are working in harmony, as a team, supporting her and her family with clear patterns of referral and a smooth transfer of information and responsibility.

1.6   Antenatal care should take place as far as is practicable in the local community, with ready access to specialised advice should it be necessary. The woman should feel confident that the antenatal consultations have a specific purpose, and that any tests and investigations have a clearly defined and valid objective, relevant to her particular circumstances.

1.7   Throughout pregnancy the woman and her partner should be encouraged to explore the possibilities for the birth itself. This may be done at antenatal groups and drop-in sessions, and then discussed more fully with her midwife or doctor.

1.8   The woman should be able to make her decisions about the plan for birth when she is ready. She should not feel that she is being rushed into an early decision. If a woman decides later in pregnancy that she wishes to change her mind about her plan, for example whether to have a hospital or home birth, this should be discussed with her in a supportive way.

1.9   The woman should feel secure in the knowledge that she can make her choice after full discussion of all the issues with the professionals involved in her care. She should also feel confident that these professionals will respect her right to choose her care on that basis, and ensure that the services provided are of the best quality possible.

1.10   Throughout her pregnancy, and most particularly during labour, the woman should be cared for by people who are familiar to her and aware of her plans for delivery. Wherever the woman has her baby, and regardless of the complications and risks that may be apparent or anticipated, the woman's care should be planned on an individual basis, and all procedures and interventions discussed and agreed with her.

1.11   During labour, the woman should feel that her psychological and physical needs are understood, her privacy is being maintained and her autonomy respected. For women who choose to give birth in hospital, the delivery suite atmosphere and environment should be supportive and welcoming as well as comfortable for the woman and her companion. This will be achieved in part by the physical surroundings, but most importantly, by the staff who are providing care.

1.12   Following the birth the woman and her partner, if present, should be left to relax with their new baby, confident in the knowledge that help and advice are readily available.

1.13   In the early days and weeks following the delivery the woman and her partner should feel assured that support and expertise are readily available to them and their baby. If the birth took place in hospital the woman should return home fully aware of the ways in which she can ask for and receive support from the midwife, the general practitioner, and the health visitor, for herself and her family.

The Group believes that this good practice can become standard practice. In some places it is already well under way. The speed with which it can be achieved will vary depending in part on the drive and enthusiasm of purchasers, providers and users but will also be affected by the complexity of the population served. We do not underestimate the challenges that can be encountered in areas of diverse social, cultural and ethnic backgrounds. But we have been heartened by the evidence we have seen that it is sometimes from within such areas that the most innovative and progressive schemes emerge.

We are confident that this vision of future services will be accepted and supported by professionals, consumer organisations and, most importantly, the women themselves.

The sections that follow identify the three key principles which the Expert Group believes should be the foundations for a woman centred service, together with points for action to help achieve this.

Principles of Good Maternity Care

The woman must be the focus of maternity care. She should be able to feel that she is in control of what is happening to her and able to make decisions about her care, based on her needs, having discussed matters fully with the professionals involved.

Maternity services must be readily and easily accessible to all. They should be sensitive to the needs of the local population and based primarily in the community.

Women should be involved in the monitoring and planning of maternity services to ensure that they are responsive to the needs of a changing society. In addition care should be effective and resources used efficiently.

2 *Appropriate Care*

The Expert Maternity Group believes that the first principle of the maternity services should be:

"The woman must be the focus of maternity care. She should be able to feel that she is in control of what is happening to her and able to make decisions about her care, based on her needs, having discussed matters fully with the professionals involved."

For every woman, pregnancy and birth are a unique experience. For some women, supported by family and friends, it will be a time of great happiness and fulfilment. Pregnancy will progress smoothly to the birth of a healthy and much welcomed baby. For others this will not be the case. The pregnancy may not be planned, complications may occur or social circumstances may be adverse. The birth itself may be complicated and the outcome different from the one anticipated or hoped for.

2.1   Safety

2.1.1   In much of the evidence received by the Group there was a strong emphasis on the need to ensure that care was designed around the needs of the individual woman and the choices she may wish to make. The issue of safety in relation to choice surfaced often during our Group's discussions. It was clear that this is a complex area, and before discussing appropriate care, it has been thought right to explore this issue.

2.1.2   Safety is an underlying principle of the maternity services. No-one cares more about achieving a safe and happy outcome to a pregnancy than the pregnant woman and her partner. Women want healthy babies and also to be healthy themselves after they have given birth. But this incorporates their desire to experience pregnancy, childbirth and the early days of parenthood as positive and fulfilling. Professionals working within the maternity services share this aim.

2.1.3   The issue of safety, however, used as an over-riding principle, may become an excuse for unnecessary interventions and technological surveillance which detract from the experience of the mother. It has to be acknowledged that some of the interventions of recent years, for example electronic fetal heart monitoring, have gained acceptance because of the assumption that they would increase the likelihood of a safe outcome. It is important that benefits are proven rather than assumed.

2.1.4   Although a good outcome to a pregnancy is desired by the woman, her family, and the professionals who care for her, we found situations where there appeared to be a conflict. We heard that some professionals appear to believe that occasionally women seem to care more about their own wellbeing than they do about the health of their unborn child. Some mothers, on the other hand, described unsympathetic doctors and midwives who used "safety" as a reason to try to impose arrangements or interventions which the mothers found unhelpful and disturbing.

2.1.5   These examples are extreme, but from the evidence we received, may not be rare. In planning change, a way must be found to ensure that such conflict becomes a thing of the past.

2.1.6   Safety is not an absolute concept. It is part of a greater picture encompassing all aspects of health and wellbeing. Each woman should be approached as an individual, and given clear and unbiased information on the options that are available to her, and in this way helped to balance the risks and benefits for herself and her baby.

2.1.7   We believe that safety, encompassing as it does the emotional and physical wellbeing of the mother and baby, must remain the foundation of good maternity care.

2.2 Meeting the needs of individuals

2.2.1 The Expert Maternity Group's approach to safety is therefore integral to our concern that women and their families should be moved to centre-stage in the maternity services. To achieve this, the service will need to be flexible and responsive to the individual needs of families being served, and women must be able to choose who they want to provide their maternity care.

2.2.2 If women are to be given a real choice about who provides their care, they must be informed that it is possible for them to go to a midwife or their general practitioner direct, for the initial consultation about their pregnancy. Information about the ways in which local midwives can be contacted must therefore be widely available.

2.2.3 The General Medical Services Committee of the British Medical Association, the Royal College of General Practitioners and the Royal College of Midwives in their joint evidence to the Group[8] state: *"A woman may wish to refer herself directly to a midwife. In these circumstances it is essential that the midwife keeps the GP informed of her obstetric progress throughout pregnancy and the puerperium."* We fully endorse this view.

2.2.4 If a woman chooses a midwife for her maternity care, it should not preclude the woman also visiting her GP about her pregnancy. The Expert Group expects GPs and midwives to work in a complementary way and does not wish to encourage competition between the professions. The woman's choice should be respected, with the professionals involved working together to support her. Similarly, if the woman wishes to be referred to an obstetrician, her GP should arrange this for her but she should also be given the name of a midwife she can contact for advice.

2.2.5 Some women will choose to book with an obstetrician either because their GP or midwife advises it or because this is their personal preference. All women should be offered the opportunity to meet an obstetrician at least once during pregnancy.

2.2.6 At her first visit to the midwife or GP the woman should be able to discuss her views and wishes and feel confident that she will receive unbiased information about the options open to her. Where her first language is not English, interpretation facilities must be organised as early as possible and the woman given the name of a contact person who speaks her language.

2.2.7 The Expert Group heard many stories illustrating ways in which sensitive and flexible professional care can enhance the experience and safety of

---

[8] *Quality issues in maternity services - a consensus statement:* a joint paper produced by the General Medical Services Committee, the Royal College of General Practitioners and the Royal College of Midwives, and presented as evidence to the Expert Maternity Group.

pregnancy and birth. One woman told the Group that "having a baby is such a lovely thing". As she described the skill, sensitivity and kind attention of her midwife, it became apparent how professionals can enhance the woman's experience by meeting her needs and leaving her with positive memories of the birth of her baby.

2.2.8 However another woman described an apparently small incident but to her it typified a regimented kind of care which appeared to focus on rules and control. Although these rules may have had a sound basis, the woman and her partner could not see a rationale for them. The woman had wished to drink apple juice while she was in labour, and had brought some cartons to the hospital with her. The midwife caring for her forbade her to drink the juice. There was no discussion or justification for the decision.

2.2.9 The attitude of professionals can influence mothers' perceptions, experience and memories of the birth. Services can be reorganised, roles and responsibilities altered, but we are convinced that the most fundamental change that needs to occur is one of attitude on the part of some care-givers.

2.2.10 Changing attitudes is not easy, but there are many instances where this has already been achieved. When it was first suggested that women should hold their own notes there was strong resistance from some doctors and midwives. As time has passed attitudes have changed and it is now becoming normal practice. The evidence on this issue suggests that when a woman is able to hold her own case notes she has a stronger sense of control[9]. This sense of control may be as a result of the woman feeling better informed and therefore more able to be fully involved in discussions about her care, and able to ask questions about what is recorded in the notes.

2.2.11 When planning care it should be remembered that for the majority of women, pregnancy and birth will be uncomplicated. However there are women who will, despite their apparently uncomplicated status, develop problems during pregnancy or labour. So whoever is caring for the woman must ensure that problems are recognised early and referrals made promptly. This is most likely to work smoothly and efficiently where GPs, obstetricians and midwives have established good working relationships based on mutual respect.

2.2.12 Professionals should be able to identify women who need less intensive monitoring and intervention during pregnancy and labour. Whenever possible, the physiological processes should be supported for all births. The

[9]Hodnett E D. *Women carrying their own case-notes during pregnancy.* In: Pregnancy and Childbirth Module, Cochrane Database of Systematic Reviews: review No. 03776, 27 April 1993. Published through Cochrane Updates on Disk, Oxford: Update Software Ltd, Spring 1993.

principle of justifying any tests and the use of technology should apply in all situations.

2.2.13 Even where a pregnancy is complicated, the woman should be fully informed and involved in making decisions about her care. There is considerable evidence that, even when the pregnancy or birth becomes highly complicated, if the woman feels in control she will feel greater satisfaction at the end of the process[10].

2.2.14 We believe that to a great extent appropriate care can be enhanced through a one-to-one relationship with a named professional within the service. The provision of a known and trusted professional for every woman in pregnancy is a central part of flexible and personal care.

2.2.15 The Group recognises that there will always be occasions when, for some reason, the relationship between the woman and the person providing care is less than satisfactory. In these circumstances, it should be possible, with the woman's agreement, for another professional to be designated. The information provided to a pregnant woman at the beginning of her pregnancy should advise her who she should contact if she is having difficulties with the professional responsible for her care.

OBJECTIVE

Women should be fully involved when decisions are to be made about their care. They should have a choice regarding the professional who will lead their care and should, if they wish, carry their own case notes. They should be kept fully informed on matters relating to their care.

ACTION POINTS

<u>Purchasers</u> should ensure that providers are achieving these objectives through the contracting and monitoring process.

<u>Providers</u> should:

* ensure that the services of a midwife are readily accessible to women when they first seek care;

* make the necessary arrangements to ensure that all women are able to carry their case notes if they wish; and

* ensure that women are fully informed on matters relating to their care and are fully involved when decisions are to be made about their care.

---

[10] Green, JM; Coupland VA, Kitzinger JB. *Expectations, experiences and psychological outcomes of childbirth: a prospective study of 825 women.* Births March 1990; Volume 17: pp15-24.

2.3 Trusted and familiar faces

2.3.1 When a woman is having a baby, nothing can replace the support of a known and trusted professional. Many women described to the Group the reassurance of seeing a familiar face at critical points, when they were anxious or when complications arose, but especially when they went into labour. They described the importance of being able to develop a relationship of trust, with "my midwife" or "my doctor", someone who is familiar with their antenatal history and their plans for the birth.

2.3.2 The evidence from the Royal College of Midwives, the Royal College of Obstetricians and Gynaecologists, the Royal College of Anaesthetists, the National Childbirth Trust, the Association for Improvements in the Maternity Services, the Maternity Alliance and other groups all expressed the same view about this subject. Continuity of carer is seen as being one of the fundamental principles underpinning woman centred care.

2.3.3 One of the requirements of the Patient's Charter is the provision of a named midwife for every woman who is having maternity care. As soon as practicable, but at least by the second visit, a woman should be given the name of her midwife. The Charter requires that this midwife be responsible for the provision of midwifery care to the woman, and in this way continuity of carer should be improved.

2.3.4 Wherever possible the named midwife should be located in the community. This neighbourhood midwife should feel comfortable practising both in the community and the hospital. The principle that the midwife should be with the woman when and where she is needed is of crucial importance.

2.3.5 The Government's response to the Health Committee report highlighted the need for a lead professional to be identified for each woman. We endorse this view. The woman should be included in discussions about who is to be her lead professional, and her view should be taken into account. In many instances, the named midwife can be the lead professional.

2.3.6 In other instances, normally when the pregnancy is more complicated, the obstetrician will be the lead professional. Some women, with uncomplicated pregnancies, may prefer to have an obstetrician or their GP take this role. Liaison between the named midwife and the lead professional is clearly essential in these circumstances.

2.3.7 The Institute of Manpower Studies (IMS) Report *Mapping Team Midwifery*,[11] which was studied by the Expert Group, shows the degree of commitment that professionals have to changing the way in which they

---

[11] *Mapping Team Midwifery.* Institute of Manpower Studies. IMS Report series 242. March 1993.

work in order to improve continuity of carer. Over 40% of units reported that they had tried to implement team midwifery. We noted, however, that very few of the schemes had managed to achieve continuity of carer in the terms set out by the IMS Team. These were that:

- the team should have no more than 6 midwives;

- each team should have a defined caseload and provide total care;

- 50% or more of women should have their baby delivered by a midwife known to her; and

- there should be teamwork in all areas according to client need.

2.3.8   Some providers have tried to achieve continuity of carer through "domino" schemes, the creation of team midwifery or midwife group practices. Some of these developments will need further refinement and evaluation if they are to achieve their aim.

2.3.9   The Group found that many teams were too large to provide continuity, and in some the midwives worked either in the hospital or in the community. In most maternity units there was an attempt to develop a cohesive philosophy of care, but from the woman's viewpoint this was no substitute for a known and trusted professional supporting her throughout pregnancy, labour and the postnatal period.

2.3.10   On visits, we noted that with the introduction of the "team" concept, some of the stronger aspects of pre-existing schemes had been lost. This was particularly obvious in antenatal care. In some cases, where the woman had previously been cared for by her general practitioner and a midwife who regularly attended that clinic, the introduction of team midwifery could lead to her meeting up to eight midwives during her pregnancy as well as her general practitioner. While some people may argue that this is a price worth paying, provided that the woman is delivered by one of those midwives, it is clear that the advantages of having one or two people to provide antenatal care for the woman are lost.

2.3.11   We were particularly impressed by the way team midwifery was working in Scunthorpe. In this unit, the changes were carefully planned, clear objectives were set, and the results are being monitored to ensure that the intended aims are being achieved.

2.3.12   The Group also heard and discussed evidence about midwifery group practices which aim to provide a high degree of support and continuity, mainly through a single midwife for each woman. These appear to demonstrate high quality practice and the most complete continuity of carer.

2.3.13   However, they exist in only small numbers, operating largely outside the NHS in the independent sector, and are not yet proven as a practical model on the large scale necessary to ensure significant success and impact nationally. In particular their costs may be rather higher than traditional arrangements. There are, however, many new employment opportunities being explored within the NHS and a more flexible approach, with a more professional pay structure, may achieve the desired changes within budget. The Group would like to see some experimental schemes being introduced within the NHS in the next five years.

2.3.14   Making continuity of carer a reality will require a substantial degree of flexibility from midwives and their managers. Some midwives will welcome the opportunity to develop their skills more fully, and will be able to adjust their personal lives so that they can be available when a woman needs them. For other midwives this will not be the case. Providers will need to acknowledge that as midwives accept more responsibility, their terms of employment, including remuneration, may need to be reviewed.

2.3.15   The need to achieve continuity of carer should not be related only to midwives. Some women told members of the Group that they had never met the consultant whose name was on their case notes. This is undesirable, both for the women and for the consultants involved. As midwives take more responsibility for caring for women with uncomplicated pregnancies, obstetricians should have more time to care for those women whose pregnancies are complicated. This should improve the quality of obstetric consultations and also facilitate continuity of carer.

2.3.16   Evidence from the MORI poll suggests that the greatest continuity is currently being provided by GPs. Where GPs are providing continuity of carer throughout the pregnancy, birth and postnatal period we were told by a number of women how much they appreciated their family doctor's involvement. The Group recommends that GPs should be encouraged to develop the skills and experience to enable them to continue their involvement in the intrapartum period.

2.3.17   The Group is aware that achieving continuity of carer will require commitment and a considerable amount of planning. Each maternity unit will need to seek its own models and strategies for achieving this aim, working in close liaison with purchasers, family health services authorities and consumers.

2.3.18   There is considerable empirical evidence to suggest that the constant presence of a trained care-giver, reassurance and a comforting touch in labour will have a positive effect on the physical and psychological outcome. We believe that the aims of the service should be for every woman to have a midwife with her throughout her labour, if she wishes. If possible, the same midwife should remain with the woman throughout.

OBJECTIVE

Every woman should have the name of a midwife who works locally, is known to her, and whom she can contact for advice. She should also know the name of the lead professional who is responsible for planning and monitoring her care. Within 5 years, 75% of women should be cared for in labour by a midwife whom they have come to know during pregnancy.

ACTION POINTS

<u>Purchasers and providers</u> should develop a strategy which ensures that:

* the named midwife and lead professional concepts are fully implemented within an agreed time scale; and

* progress towards these objectives is carefully monitored.

2.4 Access to maternity unit beds

2.4.1 From the evidence received, it appears that currently if a woman wishes to have her baby in a maternity unit she has to be booked with a consultant or GP willing to provide the service.

2.4.2 There is nothing in legislation to prevent midwives admitting women in labour to maternity unit beds, and local administrative arrangements should now be made to facilitate this. The maternity unit at the Royal Berkshire and Battle Hospital NHS Trust, Reading, has been working very well in this way for 9 years.

2.4.3 Access to maternity unit beds by midwives should prevent women having to visit hospital clinics in order to book with a consultant obstetrician. It will reduce the doctors' workload and increase the likelihood of continuity of carer.

2.4.4 The Expert Group believes that with woman centred care, it is the woman who will book the midwife, consultant or GP rather than, as is currently the case, the woman being booked by the professional.

OBJECTIVE

A woman with an uncomplicated pregnancy should, if she wishes, be able to book with a midwife as the lead professional for the entire episode of care including delivery in a general hospital.

ACTION POINTS

<u>Purchasers</u> **should:**

* **ensure through their service specifications that women can book with a midwife for their entire episode of care; and**

* **ensure that all women who become pregnant are informed about this option.**

<u>Providers</u> **should ensure appropriate arrangements are in place to enable a woman to book with a midwife as her lead professional for her entire episode of care, including delivery in hospital.**

2.5 Reviewing antenatal care

2.5.1 Antenatal care was the area where the Group found that services were often not focused in the most appropriate or consistent manner. In some instances decisions about tests, interventions and surveillance were arbitrary or varied between professionals.

2.5.2 In her evidence to us, a woman described how she had carefully kept a "fetal movement chart" between antenatal visits, having been told to do so by a midwife. She returned to the clinic four weeks later and showed the chart to a different midwife, who said that she did not know why the woman was told to fill it in, and that it was a waste of time. She gave no further explanation. Events like this undermine a woman's confidence and leave her concerned about the ability of the professionals who are caring for her. Consistency is important.

2.5.3 In the majority of units we visited there was a commitment to reducing the number of antenatal visits made by the woman to the hospital. In some units this had already been achieved by transferring care to community clinics. However, there did not appear to have been a fundamental reappraisal of the purpose of antenatal care, in particular the number and content of the antenatal check-ups. We welcome the move towards more antenatal care in the community, but would like to see this accompanied by a thorough review of the care given, particularly in the light of the advances being made in fetal medicine.

2.5.4 The Group saw the evidence that has been produced on the value of routine antenatal care over 10 years ago by Marion Hall and colleagues[12], which highlighted the possible over-surveillance of the woman during the antenatal period. If these checkups are unwarranted, it is not only a waste of resources, but could impact adversely on the standards that can be achieved. If fewer visits are necessary it should be easier to plan the workload of individual members of staff, to increase both the level of continuity achieved and the time spent on each visit, thereby improving the quality of care.

2.5.5 Even for women with uncomplicated pregnancies it is not uncommon for them to experience 12-14 antenatal visits. In 1982 a Working Party of the Royal College of Obstetricians and Gynaecologists (RCOG) on Antenatal and Intrapartum Care[13] recommended a pattern of 9 visits for primigravidae and 6 otherwise. On conservative estimates this could have reduced the workload by 25% in the antenatal clinic of a maternity unit

[12]Hall M H, Chng P K, MacGillivray I. *Is routine antenatal care worthwhile?* Lancet, 12 July 1980: pp 78 -80

[13]Report of the RCOG Working Party on Antenatal and Intrapartum Care. Royal College of Obstetricians and Gynaecologists: September 1982; Appendix 2.

19

with 3,500 births per year. On our visits we saw little evidence that those recommendations had been implemented. While there have been changes in maternity care in the past decade we believe that the recommendations made by the RCOG are still valid. If the changes were implemented, the time saved could then be used to improve the quality of the remaining visits and to facilitate some of the changes in practice that will be necessary to move towards more community or home-based services.

2.5.6   The system of antenatal care currently in place is cumbersome and a source of concern to professionals and pregnant women alike. The Expert Group strongly recommends that a survey of existing practice is undertaken by purchasers, providers and professionals on a regular basis. As well as reviewing the number of antenatal check-ups the effectiveness of the service in identifying the fetus at risk should also be assessed. Streamlining the current system could achieve improvement for all involved.

2.5.7   We recognise that some women, used to more traditional antenatal visiting patterns, may feel anxious if they hear of plans to reduce the number of visits. Time should be taken to explain that a reduction in antenatal visits will not mean any less support during pregnancy, but rather that the quality and continuity of the care will be improved, and waiting times reduced. The woman should know that she can telephone her midwife if she has any anxieties or worries between check-ups.

2.5.8   Parent education sessions and drop-in groups can provide a very useful source of support to women and their partners during pregnancy, and sometimes following the birth of the baby. A variety of approaches can help. For example, Norfolk and Norwich Hospital parent education department has developed a wide range of groups for women and couples with common interests. There are "solo" groups for teenagers without a partner, sessions for parents who are going to adopt a baby, and refresher groups for women who have attended before, as well as a comprehensive programme for first time parents.

2.5.9   Women tend most often to seek advice from their family and friends. It should not be surprising that they too wish to be up-to-date and informed about current thinking in the care of newborn babies. In Scunthorpe, in response to an increasing number of requests, the midwives ran some sessions for grandparents. These have been well attended. The content of the session is determined by those who attend, but there is a consistent interest in infant feeding and cot death.

2.5.10 Many women and their partners find these groups valuable, giving them the opportunity to explore the realities of life following the birth of their new babies. Providers need to ensure that the approach is tailored around the views of the client group. The National Childbirth Trust offers one model, and pregnancy clubs and drop-in centres, examples of which are described in Part II of *Changing Childbirth*, provide others. As with all aspects of maternity care, purchasers and providers should identify needs in this area, plan appropriately with users, and review the outcome.

2.5.11   Another aspect of the care and support that can be required in pregnancy is in relation to screening for fetal abnormality. A wide range of tests and investigations is now available, and it is often at the first visit that a woman and her partner are expected to make decisions about the tests they will wish to have.

2.5.12   We were told that sometimes, due to the rushed nature of the first consultation, women can feel as if the whole episode is focused on the screening tests that are available. It is essential that women are given sufficient information and proper counselling on these issues.

2.5.13   We are aware that some professionals have produced excellent information material on screening. For example, we were shown a carefully-made video produced by Professor John Burn of the Clinical Genetics Department in Newcastle-upon-Tyne which deals with the issue of maternal serum screening for Down's Syndrome. Purchasers and providers should make use of the available materials. They should also consider commissioning or making material of their own if they identify areas where women's needs are not being met.

2.5.14   The need to prevent unnecessary admission of pregnant women to hospital is well accepted. In many of the units we visited, antenatal day assessment units (or fetal assessment units) had been established. The rationale for these units appeared to be to reduce the number of antenatal admissions by providing tests, investigations and results on an out-patient basis. The Group had concerns about these units. In some instances the reduction in the number of antenatal admissions appeared to be minimal. The range of tests offered in the units varied tremendously, although all claimed success in identifying babies at risk. The place of antenatal assessment units has not, as yet, been properly evaluated. The growth of these units needs to be monitored, and their contribution to efficiency and effectiveness assessed before new ones are commissioned.

OBJECTIVE

Antenatal care should be provided so as to maximise the use of resources. It should also ensure that the woman and her partner feel supported and fully informed throughout the pregnancy, and are prepared for the birth and the care of their baby.

ACTION POINTS

<u>Purchasers</u> should agree a timetable for a review of antenatal care with the providers and monitor whether that timetable is being achieved.

<u>Providers</u> should:

* review the pattern of antenatal care in the light of current evidence;

* where they exist, establish clear objectives for antenatal assessment units and evaluate whether these objectives are being achieved;

* undertake a full review of parent education sessions and if necessary develop a strategy for change; and

* review the counselling arrangements for prenatal screening tests.

2.6 Place of birth

2.6.1   It was apparent to the Group that most women were given little choice about the place of birth. A MORI survey of women who had recently given birth found hospital delivery in consultant units was the only option explained fully to most of them. 98% of women in this country give birth in consultant hospital units yet nearly three quarters – 72% – would have liked at least the option of a different system of care and delivery. Of those who wanted an alternative option, 22% said they would like the choice of a home birth and 44% a midwife-led domino delivery.

2.6.2   Professionals providing care assumed that women would wish to go into hospital. Many professionals still feel that birth in a general hospital maternity unit is preferable, because of safety factors, to delivery at home or in a midwife-/GP-led unit at some distance from a general hospital.

2.6.3   Whether a mother with an uncomplicated pregnancy is putting herself and her child at any greater risk by choosing to have her baby away from a general hospital maternity unit is a topic that has been argued with vehemence and emotion for decades. The inability to reach agreement after this length of time suggests that there is no clear answer. Furthermore, professionals cannot quantify the enriching experience which some women feel when they have their baby in a place of their choice. The job of midwives and doctors, therefore, must be to provide the woman with as much accurate and objective information as possible, while avoiding personal bias or preference.

2.6.4   Women who wish to have a home birth frequently report either a lack of interest, or hostility, from the professionals they encounter[14]. The Expert Group heard accounts of some GPs who asked women and their families to transfer to another GP's list if the woman wished to have a home birth. This is clearly a distressing experience for the women and families concerned. It is an unacceptable practice which must cease. GPs who feel unable to offer care or support to a woman who wishes to have a home birth should refer the woman directly to a midwife for advice.

2.6.5   Some GPs seem reluctant to refer women to midwife-/GP-led units. From the evidence we received the Group believes that many of these units are under-used. If they are to remain viable it is essential that women are informed when this option is open to them.

2.6.6   There is no clear statistical evidence that having their babies away from general hospital maternity units is less safe for women with uncomplicated

[14] *National Childbirth Trust Maternity Services Survey. April 1991.*

pregnancies.[15] It is unlikely that it will ever be possible to know whether there is any difference in mortality: the perinatal mortality rate is now so low, and the numbers required to achieve a satisfactory sample size to detect a difference within comparable groups in a randomised trial would be prohibitively high. It is increasingly important to continue to monitor other outcomes as well as mortality.

2.6.7   A woman should be given the opportunity to discuss at her first appointment where she would like her baby to be born. But she should not be made to feel that she has to decide at that time. The majority of women will probably feel happiest deciding before labour begins. However, the Group learnt that in the Isle of Sheppey in the Medway District, women could decide at the beginning of labour whether to have their babies at home or in hospital. These women had previously discussed the possibility of a home birth or a "domino" delivery with the midwife. Having agreed that either of these options were suitable, the women sometimes made their final decision at the onset of labour. If labour then progressed smoothly the woman remained at home, otherwise she transferred to hospital.

2.6.8   The woman should be given information about the facilities and back-up that will be available to her, wherever she chooses to give birth. This should highlight the benefits and limitations of all the available options. Professionals may wish to add that, for example, that birth planned away from a general hospital may result in the woman having to undertake an uncomfortable and potentially worrying journey when she is in advanced labour if complications occur. However, it would be equally necessary to point out the evidence that for comparable groups of women, delivery in consultant maternity units within a general hospital can result in more interventions.[16]

2.6.9   From the evidence received, it is clear that the concept originally encapsulated in the "domino" scheme is very attractive to many women and professionals. Community based care and continuity of carer should ensure that the strengths associated with the scheme become features of the care received by women. They will be cared for in the community by a midwife they know, will normally be attended by her when in labour, and will return home as soon as they feel ready.

[15] *Where to be Born? The debate and the evidence.* Campbell and Macfarlane. NPEU. 1987. (Second Edition in press.).

[16] Klein M, Lloyd I, Redman C, Bull M, Turnbull AC: *A comparison of low-risk pregnant women booked for delivery in two systems of care.* Br J Obstet Gynaecol 1983; Vol 90: pp 118-122.
Lowe SW, House W, Garrett T; *A comparison of outcome of low-risk labour in an isolated general practitioner maternity unit and a specialist maternity hospital.* J RCGP 1987; Vol 37: pp 484-487.
Shearer JML: A *five-year prospective survey of risk of booking for a home birth.* BMJ 1985; Vol 291: pp 1478-1480.

2.6.10 When reviewing the available options, purchasers and providers should consider establishing a midwife-/GP-led maternity service alongside the specialist facility. This has been achieved very successfully at the Leicester Royal Infirmary NHS Trust. The unit provides a welcoming and relaxed environment for women with uncomplicated pregnancies, with specialist referral and assistance immediately available if required.

OBJECTIVE

Women should receive clear, unbiased advice and be able to choose where they would like their baby to be born. Their right to make that choice should be respected and every practical effort made to achieve the outcome that the woman believes is best for her baby and herself.

ACTION POINTS

<u>Purchasers</u> should

*   as part of their strategic plan, review the current choices available to women regarding the place of birth. Following consultation, these should be developed as appropriate for their locality and ensure that home birth is a real option for the women who may wish to have it; and

*   ensure that women receive information about the full range of options for place of birth available in her locality.

<u>Providers</u> should:

*   review their current organisation and practices to ensure that real choice about the place of birth is available; and

*   develop a flexible system of care so that women are able to take time in making their decision regarding the place of birth, and can alter that decision close to the time of birth if they so wish.

2.7   Emergency services

2.7.1   When discussing place of birth, most professionals and mothers seemed to feel that giving birth at home or in a rural midwife/GP unit is fine provided that all goes well. There is a clear perception that in the event of complications the emergency services and appropriately-trained personnel are not as readily to hand as they would be within a general hospital. This view was supported by the findings of the MORI survey.

2.7.2   This view assumes that experienced personnel are always readily available within a general hospital. We heard that on some occasions when a midwife calls for help, even within a teaching unit, the person responding may be an inexperienced senior house officer in obstetrics or paediatrics, who is clearly unable to deal with the emergency.

2.7.3   Providers must ensure that this ceases. The 1985-87 Report on Confidential Enquiries into Maternal Deaths[17] states that: "*The management of many obstetric emergencies requires experience that is only available at consultant level*", and this experience should always be available to a midwife. The role of the senior house officer in obstetrics and paediatrics needs to be defined and clear to all working in the unit. This is dealt with in more detail in section 2.13.

2.7.4   A woman giving birth at home or in a midwife/GP unit away from a general hospital should feel confident that the midwife and doctor, if present, is able to provide help efficiently and effectively in an acute emergency prior to the transfer of the mother and baby to the general hospital.

2.7.5   Back-up emergency services in the community need to be of the highest quality which is practicable. There has been a major reduction in the number of obstetric flying squads in operation in recent years. It is essential that a comprehensive review of the system for dealing with emergencies is undertaken in every health district and local procedures put into place.

2.7.6   We recommend that each district's emergency ambulance crews should be trained in the administration of intravenous fluids and be ready to provide such assistance as necessary to the midwife during the woman's transfer to hospital when a complication has occurred. A nationally agreed syllabus for obstetric training is now incorporated in the NHS Training Directorate Manual.

2.7.7   Where careful selection procedures are in place for deliveries to be undertaken at home or in rural units the risks to term babies are extremely

[17]Report on Confidential Enquiries into Maternal Deaths in the United Kingdom 1985-87. UK Health Departments 1991.

small, with no more than 2 out of every 1000 term babies requiring more than simple resuscitation.[18] A professional present at the birth who has received training and gained experience in resuscitation techniques could expect to provide appropriate resuscitation in 99% of term deliveries for which this is necessary.

2.7.8   We recommend that clear guidelines are drawn up and agreed for neonatal emergencies occurring in the community. These should cover immediate care and transfer to the neonatal unit. The requirements for that service have been clearly identified in the recent report of a British Paediatric Association Working Party on Neonatal Resuscitation.[18] A summary of the report's recommendations is at Annex 5 to this report.

2.7.9   For home births or births in midwife/GP units, ideally two professionals, two midwives or a GP and midwife, should be present at the birth so that one is free to provide resuscitation if necessary. Implicit in this statement is that those professionals present at the birth must be trained and practised in neonatal resuscitation.

2.7.10   The responsibilities accepted by midwives in caring for women who wish to have a home birth must be acknowledged. Obstetricians and GPs should ensure that they support the midwives, and that they make clear their readiness to give advice and help if needed.

---

[18] *Neonatal Resuscitation: The Report of a British Paediatric Association Working Party.* June 1993.

OBJECTIVE

When emergency services are required by the woman or her baby at, or around, the time of birth, they should be of the highest standard that can be achieved in the circumstances.

ACTION POINTS

<u>Purchasers</u> should agree a timetable with ambulance services for the target of one paramedic on each frontline ambulance able to offer appropriate support to the midwife in caring for the woman in an emergency.

<u>Providers</u> should:

* review procedures for dealing with emergencies, including lines of communication;

* establish a formal ongoing staff training and updating programme dealing with common neonatal emergency procedures taking account of the guidance available in the British Paediatric Association Working Party Report on Neonatal Resuscitation; and

* ensure that consultant obstetricians are prepared to offer advice and as much support as is practicable to midwives undertaking home births. This is in addition to the support already provided by the local supervisor of midwives.

2.8 Care in labour

2.8.1 *"It is easy in the hospital atmosphere of professional childbirth to forget how terrifying childbirth often is, especially to the inexperienced young mother, and how much the patient can be comforted and soothed by gentleness and consideration, and a little time spent explaining away anxiety or fear. A placid patient is so much more likely to have an easy delivery than one who is frightened or over-strained that such attention is part of good midwifery practice as well as of humane care."* Dame Janet Campbell 1935[19].

2.8.2 While the care of women in labour may, in some ways, have changed a great deal in the intervening 60 years, the sentiments expressed by Dame Janet Campbell are as relevant today, when 99% of births occur in maternity units, as they were to the audience she addressed all those years ago.

2.8.3 The midwife and doctor should be able to discuss any questions or anxieties that the woman may have about labour when she has her antenatal check-up. Parent education groups should also give women the opportunity to discuss and learn about labour and birth, and to explore the approaches that will be available to them.

2.8.4 It is important that the woman's plans and wishes about the birth of her baby are documented in her maternity notes. A birth plan may be used for this purpose, either incorporated in advance into the notes or supplied by the woman herself. Birth plans should not just be for women who have unusual requests. Birth is a unique experience for every woman, and if, unavoidably, the woman is cared for in labour by someone whom she has not met, the birth plan will be particularly helpful.

2.8.5 On visits, the Group was impressed by the degree of flexibility expressed by some professionals involved in maternity care, particularly about care in labour. In many places, there was an interest in different approaches, and midwives and doctors seemed keen to ensure that the woman's experience matched her expectations as closely as possible.

2.8.6 From the evidence presented to us by the National Childbirth Trust, it was apparent that some women still find professionals unhelpful and resistant to new ideas. The woman may find it extremely difficult trying to negotiate with the professionals who will ultimately be providing her care. Professionals should be open to discussion and thereby encourage women to express their views and expectations regarding labour. In the vast majority of cases it is possible to accommodate the woman's wishes provided those involved are prepared to be flexible.

---

[19]*Maternity Services.* Dame Janet Campbell. Faber and Faber. 1935.

2.8.7   The environment in which the birth takes place is important to a woman and her partner, and it should be as supportive and comfortable as possible. If the birth takes place in hospital, the beds in the delivery suites should be comfortable for the woman, and she should be free to move around and adopt new positions as labour progresses. On visits it was obvious to us that relatively minor changes in delivery rooms could enhance the environment considerably. Moving the bed to one side, removing unnecessary equipment, and using subdued lighting all seemed to have a significant impact. It is also essential that the privacy of the woman and her partner is respected and that they are not subjected to unnecessary interruptions.

2.8.8   Being cared for in labour by a midwife whom she knows, may be reassuring to a woman and reduce her need for pharmacological pain relief. This view was expressed by representatives of the Royal College of Anaesthetists when they gave evidence to the Group, reinforcing yet again the need to achieve continuity of carer.

2.8.9   The contribution made by obstetric anaesthetists has substantially changed childbirth for many women in this country. For women who wish to have a pain-free labour, epidural analgesia seems the ideal choice. Anaesthetists told us that they would welcome the opportunity to meet women before labour begins to explain the options that are available to them. For women who wish to have an epidural, or who wish to discuss the idea more fully, this would obviously be an advantage. Early discussions with an anaesthetist would also be beneficial for any woman with medical problems or obstetric complications which might limit the choice of methods of pain relief or types of anaesthesia for operative delivery.

2.8.10   Obstetric anaesthesia has also had a very positive impact for women who need to have an operative delivery. Epidural anaesthesia can allow a woman, if she wishes, to remain fully conscious and aware during her baby's birth, even when delivered by caesarian section. Moreover it can be a safer option than general anaesthesia.[20]

2.8.11   Anaesthetists also have a crucial role to play in the care of some women who become acutely ill in pregnancy, labour and following the birth. To minimise mortality and ill-health it is essential that anaesthetists are involved as early as possible when these complications occur or are anticipated.

2.8.12   The support of the paediatric team is often required on the delivery suite. In some instances it will be evident in advance that a baby will need extra care and support. If at all possible, the parents should have the opportunity

[20]Report on Confidential Enquiries into Maternal Deaths in England and Wales 1982 - 84. Department of Health, 1989.

to meet the paediatricians and visit the neonatal unit before the birth. To minimise delay, there should always be clear guidelines for obtaining paediatric support during or following the birth.

2.8.13　Even with the best care and support there will still be occasions when a baby is stillborn or dies shortly after birth. We recognise the progress that has been made in helping staff to help parents and their families at this very difficult time, but in some units there may still be a need for further training of staff in this sensitive issue. The Stillbirth and Neonatal Death Society's booklet, *Miscarriage, Stillbirth and Neonatal death: Guidelines for Professionals*[21], gives excellent advice on this difficult subject and should be readily available in every maternity unit.

2.8.14　Birth is normally a time of great happiness for a woman and her family. The contribution of midwives and doctors should enhance this by providing low-key support when all is going well, complemented by more sophisticated care when complications occur.

OBJECTIVE

Women should have the opportunity to discuss their plans for labour and birth. Their decisions should be recorded in their birth plans and incorporated into their case notes. Every reasonable effort should be made to accommodate the wishes of the woman and her partner, and to inform them of the services that are available to them.

ACTION POINTS

Purchasers should:

*　**use service specifications to ensure that the care of a woman in labour is flexible and able to accommodate the woman's individual needs and preferences; and**

*　**assess whether the target is being achieved by auditing consumer satisfaction.**

Providers should:

*　**ensure that women have the opportunity to explore and discuss their wishes regarding labour and birth with a midwife or obstetrician;**

*　**ensure that the woman's wishes are recorded in her birth plan; and**

*　**have agreed guidelines for the care of women in labour which include guidance on obtaining anaesthetic and paediatric advice.**

---

[21] *Miscarriage, Stillbirth and Neonatal Death: Guidelines for Professionals.* Stillbirth and Neonatal Death Society. 1991.

2.9 Postnatal care

2.9.1 The needs of each woman and her baby will differ in the postnatal period as will the support they require. The care offered must be flexible, but the woman and her family must be confident that the professional expertise and help of the named midwife is readily available to them at home or in the hospital.

2.9.2 If the birth takes place in hospital, the new parents must be given the opportunity to get to know their new baby on their own. At the same time, the woman should know how to obtain help or advice if she feels that she needs it.

2.9.3 As far as practicable, the length of time spent in a postnatal ward should be discussed and agreed between the woman, the midwife and other professionals as necessary. The midwife can help the woman to assess her readiness to return home and to prepare her for doing so.

2.9.4 For some women, after the first few days at home, it will be enough to know that they can contact their midwife for advice or a visit if they are concerned about themselves or their babies. For others, the visits of a familiar midwife, and their GP, in the period up to 28 days after the birth of their babies will be essential to build confidence in their own abilities. Patterns of care must also provide for a smooth transition from the care of midwives to health visitors. It will usually be appropriate to discuss with the mother how and when, within the 10-28 day period, she would prefer the transfer of main support from the midwife to her health visitor to take place.

2.9.5 On some occasions, midwives will have concerns about the health of the baby. While she would normally call the GP in these circumstances, it should also be possible for her, if she considers it necessary, to refer immediately to a paediatrician. We are aware that this facility is available in some health districts and would welcome similar developments elsewhere.

2.9.6 Mothers and babies should not be separated unless this is absolutely necessary for the care of either: frequent contact between babies and their parents is an essential part of their development and their well-being. This is equally the case when either the baby or the mother are ill. Every effort should be made to ensure that babies receive an appropriate level of care and that only babies who need continuous medical and nursing supervision receive it in a neonatal unit. In the event of a multiple birth, every attempt should be made to keep the babies together.

2.9.7 Babies who are ill should be cared for in a local unit as near as possible to their parents. While every maternity unit should be able to meet the immediate needs of most babies and mothers, there will inevitably be occasions when care has to be provided elsewhere. There should be clear guidelines in place for babies and mothers to be transferred to units which have the necessary facilities and expertise. In arranging transfers to other units, sensitivity should be accorded to the needs of both babies and parents in terms of visiting and distance of the unit from their homes. At such a difficult time for parents and families, strenuous efforts must be made to involve them in decisions and ensure that they are given full explanations of the arrangements for transfer.

2.9.8   The support of a midwife that a woman knows during her pregnancy should enhance a woman's confidence about asking for advice in the time immediately following birth. We noted the results of the 1990 OPCS Survey of Infant Feeding[22] which indicated that there had been no improvement in recent years in the number of women who successfully breastfeed their babies. If women can ask for help from someone they know and trust, this situation might be improved.

2.9.9   A woman who is feeding her baby confidently is less likely to feel insecure and anxious. It is important that professionals listen to the anxieties and worries that women have about feeding, whichever method is used, and advise and encourage them as needed, ensuring that the advice given is consistent and does not conflict with that given by other professionals. Many women also receive sympathetic advice and support from voluntary breastfeeding organisations or breastfeeding counsellors.

2.9.10   The ongoing training of GPs, midwives and health visitors should include updating their knowledge about all aspects of infant nutrition.

2.9.11   Professionals need to be alert to the possibility of women developing postnatal depression. 10 – 15% of women suffer postnatal depression and 50 – 66% experience postnatal blues. The relative risk of admission to a psychiatric hospital with a psychotic illness is 22 times greater in the first month after the birth of a child than in any of the preceding two years.[23] Mental illness is one of the five key areas in the Government's strategy document *The Health of the Nation*, and the key area handbook on mental illness[24] advises that all professional groups would benefit from the development of general and specialist skills in appropriate care and treatment of postnatal depression. We strongly support this view.

---

[22] *Infant Feeding 1990*. White A, Freeth S, O'Brien M. Office of Population, Censuses and Surveys. HMSO 1992.

[23] Tilowsky L *et al* (eds) 1991. *Women and Mental Health*. Br J Psychiatry; Vol 158: Supp 10.

[24] *The Health of the Nation.. – Key Area Handbook: Mental Illness*. Department of Health. January 1993.

OBJECTIVE

A woman who gives birth in hospital should return home, as far as is practicable, when she feels ready. Once home, she should be supported by her midwife, knowing that the general practitioner is available if medical advice is necessary. The pattern of support should be appropriate to the woman's needs and planned in consultation with her.

ACTION POINTS

<u>Providers</u> should:

* have as flexible an approach as is practicable to the length of postnatal stay. This should normally be decided by the mother, following consultation with the midwife and obstetrician if appropriate;

* have a flexible approach to postnatal home visiting ensuring that the views of the woman and her family determine the level of support provided by the midwife and health visitor;

* monitor patterns of infant feeding and assess whether women are receiving appropriate information and advice, and feel confident with the method they have chosen; and

* ensure that advice from a consultant paediatrician is available to a midwife working in the community should it be required.

2.10 The role of the general practitioner

2.10.1 During the course of our visits many women told us how much they valued the involvement of their general practitioners (GPs) during their maternity care. One woman said that the fact that the GP knew her before she was pregnant and would continue to care for her and her family after the birth of her baby was very reassuring to her. The Maternity Units Study Team (MUST) report[25] acknowledged that the GP is the generalist who is able to give overall health care, often over many years and sometimes across generations.

2.10.2 GPs were involved in some way in the antenatal care of approximately 98% of the women interviewed for the MORI survey. This involvement may have been restricted to an initial consultation or may have extended to providing most of the care during pregnancy, being present during or for part of the labour, and providing support during the postnatal period.

2.10.3 Less than 6% of births (other than home births) in England and Wales take place under GP care[26], some of these occurring in rural maternity units. The Group is aware that only a very small number of GPs maintain an active interest in intrapartum care but recognise that this small group has played a crucial role in the survival of some rural units.

2.10.4 We were concerned about the evidence which we received during our visits and from research in the field that some GPs appear reluctant to refer women to midwife/GP-led units. This related both to midwife/GP-led units in general hospitals as well as those in rural areas. It became clear that the continued existence of such units is dependent on the willingness of GPs to be involved in them. The Group heard from a number of women that they themselves valued this particular option for their maternity care and we formed the view that it would be regrettable if such units were allowed to disappear.

2.10.5 We are keen to see an end to the duplication and repetition that currently occurs across the service between GPs, midwives and obstetricians. Midwives expressed concern to us that GPs receive a fee for antenatal services but that often the midwife actually provides the care. However, the fee at present paid to the GP is for ensuring that antenatal care is provided[27] – it is not for providing the care. The antenatal fee is part of the more complex fees for services arrangement of the GPs' contract.

[25] *A study of midwife- and GP-led maternity units: report of the Maternity Units Study Team.* Department of Health. January 1993.

[26] Smith LFP, Jewell D. *Contributions of the general practitioner to hospital intrapartum care in maternity units in England and Wales in 1988.* BMJ 1991; Vol 302: pp13-16.

[27] NHS (General Medical Services) Regulations 1992 Schedule 5.

2.10.6   The fee for intrapartum care is also paid on the basis that the GP has agreed to provide a service at the time he or she is needed. It does not require the GP to be present. It is beyond our remit to make specific recommendations regarding GPs' payments. However in the light of the evidence we received, the Group recommends that GPs' remuneration for maternity care should be reviewed. Any consideration should reflect the concerns which those involved in maternity care have about this matter and in particular whether the present system allows for remuneration to be targeted to those GPs who contribute substantially to maternity care. We also recommend that the obstetric list arrangements should be reviewed.

2.10.7   The number of GPs taking part in intrapartum care is falling steadily [28]. We believe that this is due to both the remuneration GPs receive for providing this service and the nature of their training. We welcome the recommendations made on the subject of training by the Royal College of Obstetricians and Gynaecologists and the Royal College of General Practitioners in their 1993 joint report on *General Practitioner Vocational Training in Obstetrics and Gynaecology.*[29]

2.10.8   There are no plans at present to include maternity care in the list of services which GP fundholders may purchase. Should this occur we would expect fundholders to ensure that women had a full range of options from which to choose.

2.10.9   Like the Select Committee, we heard of cases where GPs did not always appear to have acted in the best interests of women needing maternity care. Clearly there are some problems in this area, but many women see it as natural to turn to their GPs for care relating to their pregnancy and this option should be available to them. We believe that with the cooperation of all those involved, GPs should continue to play a valuable role in providing continuity of carer for women and their families at this very important time in their lives.

[28]See footnote to 2.10.3 above.

[29]*General Practitioner Vocational Training in Obstetrics and Gynaecology.* The Royal College of General Practitioners and the Royal College of Obstetricians and Gynaecologists 1993.

OBJECTIVE

GPs who wish to provide maternity care should receive appropriate training and encouragement to do so. Midwives and GPs should work in partnership in the best interests of the woman.

ACTION POINTS

<u>Professional and training bodies</u> should continue the development and implementation of appropriate training for GPs.

<u>The Department of Health</u> should:

*   consider with other Health Departments the need to review with the profession the current fee structure to encourage those GPs who wish to contribute substantially to maternity care; and

*   consider with other Health Departments the need to review with the profession the criteria for the inclusion of GPs on the obstetric list.

2.11 The role of the midwife

2.11.1   From the evidence we received, we recognised that women have great confidence in the midwifery profession. The midwife is able to offer a woman and her family support and encouragement during a time of great change as well as having the clinical skills necessary to determine whether all is progressing normally. Importantly, the midwife is able to work across a variety of settings, and is able to be with the woman when and where needed, ensuring that she remains the focus of care.

2.11.2   Legally, midwives are able to practise independently. When a pregnancy is uncomplicated they are able to be responsible for providing and arranging all the maternity care that is needed for a woman and her baby. If abnormalities are suspected or occur, the midwife is obliged to refer to a doctor, and to continue to provide care working with the doctor.

2.11.3   When a woman has a complicated pregnancy and books with an obstetrician, the midwife's role is to provide any additional support and advice that may be necessary.

2.11.4   In the past, changes in the organisation of maternity care have resulted in midwives working in a fragmented way, tending to specialise in particular aspects of care, rather than providing total care to a group of women.

2.11.5   In an attempt to achieve greater continuity, over 40% of maternity services have recently introduced team midwifery. The IMS study[30] found that although midwives might have been apprehensive in advance of taking up their new responsibilities and patterns of practice, once they became accustomed to the new way of working they have found it more satisfying.

2.11.6   There have been substantial changes in midwifery education over the last 10 years. All midwifery education will soon be at a minimum of diploma of higher education level and there are several undergraduate programmes of midwifery education. All courses lead to admission to part 10 of the UKCC register.

2.11.7   Midwifery education emphasises a balance of clinical skills and knowledge, the need for intellectual development, knowledge of the human sciences and the need to use scientific evidence in practice. Importantly, a high premium is placed on interpersonal and communication skills. All students are expected to become competent practising in both community and hospital before registration as a midwife.

[30] See footnote to paragraph 2.3.7

2.11.8　Midwives who have been in practice for some time without undertaking their full role may need support for professional development and in the updating of some of their skills. The Group recommends that whenever fundamental changes to the pattern of practice are planned, specific education and training needs should be identified and met.

2.11.9　With the prospect of a more community-based service, clinical accountability was an area frequently raised with the Group. We therefore sought advice from the Department of Health's solicitors, and this is reproduced in full below:

"Rule 40 of part V of the Nurses, Midwives and Health Visitors Rules 1983 imposes an obligation on the midwife to seek assistance from a registered medical practitioner where there is an emergency or where the midwife detects a deviation from the norm in the health of the mother and baby. However, if the total care remains with the midwife, and assistance has not been sought in accordance with rule 40, the midwife only would be responsible, in the event of foreseeable injury being negligently caused to either mother or baby. Even the allocation of a "named consultant" to a mother and baby does not by itself impose responsibility on the consultant for the care of that mother and baby unless the consultant has himself assumed responsibility. If the midwife failed to seek assistance when such assistance was necessary, then the responsibility for that decision rests with the midwife.

A health authority or NHS trust which employs a midwife under a contract of service would be vicariously liable for the negligence of the midwife, providing the midwife was "acting in the course of her employment". In the NHS context, the employing body will be vicariously liable whether the midwife has had total responsibility or has acted as delegate. Where the mother has herself made arrangements with a consultant or midwife for private care, liability for negligent treatment would lie, depending on the circumstances, with the consultant or with the midwife."

OBJECTIVE

The part which the midwife plays in maternity care should make full use of all her skills and knowledge, and reflect the full role for which she has been trained.

ACTION POINTS

<u>Purchasers and providers</u> should ensure that:

*　midwives' skills are fully used by developing schemes that achieve continuity of carer; and

*　there are appropriate updating programmes for midwives who are moving into new areas of practice.

2.12 The role of the obstetrician

2.12.1 Obstetricians have constantly worked to reduce maternal deaths and they were the first professionals in this country to instigate a medical audit of their work in order to improve their skill and safety record. They are acknowledged experts in the care of women with complicated pregnancies. But some obstetricians feel they do not have enough time to spend with women who have more complex needs as antenatal clinics are often overbooked and overcrowded. The Group also acknowledges that some women with uncomplicated pregnancies will choose to have an obstetrician as their lead professional and recognises that many obstetricians see providing such care as an important part of their role.

2.12.2 We hope that many obstetricians will welcome changes which ensure that they have more time to spend with women who are most in need of their care and also enhance choice for women.

2.12.3 In this changed service the role of the obstetrician will remain primarily as it is now:

* the lead professional for women with complicated pregnancies;

* an adviser on actual and suspected abnormalities;

* the person responsible for the care of women who have obstetric emergencies;

* a provider of technical skills beyond the expertise of midwives/GPs;

* fetal medicine;

* teaching junior medical staff;

* increasingly, involvement as an administrator and manager; and

* a researcher.

2.12.4 In a service in which the care of women with uncomplicated pregnancies is increasingly led by midwives, the obstetrician will have more time to concentrate on women with complicated pregnancies. But there is also a group of women who may develop complications during a previously normal pregnancy.

2.12.5 It is important that the obstetrician, midwife and the GP, keep in regular contact. Obstetricians must be involved when a problem is suspected, and not just when it has occurred. Close contact at an early stage between obstetricians, anaesthetists and paediatricians may be of great benefit to the outcome for women and their babies in the context of an imminent complicated delivery. We recommend that early consultation should take place so that the options can be considered and the best possible outcome achieved.

2.12.6   In most maternity units in the United Kingdom, teamwork involving midwives, obstetricians and paediatricians, each providing their own particular expertise, is an important feature of the service. Increasingly these professionals, in consultation with consumers, are developing guidelines to clinical practice which increase the cohesiveness of the services. It is this team work which ought to be clarified, enhanced and encouraged.

OBJECTIVE

The knowledge and skills of the obstetrician should be used primarily to provide advice, support and expertise for those women who have complicated pregnancies.

ACTION POINTS

<u>Purchasers and providers</u> should:

*   agree a strategy with obstetricians and midwives to ensure that this objective is achieved;

*   ensure that women with uncomplicated pregnancies are given the opportunity to meet a consultant obstetrician; and

*   ensure that women with uncomplicated pregnancies can choose to book with a consultant obstetrician as their lead professional, via their GP or midwife.

2.13 The role of the obstetric Senior House Officer

2.13.1 The Expert Group recognises that there is already a great deal of work under way to improve and rationalise medical training, including the proposals in the recent report by the Chief Medical Officer's working group on specialist medical training, *Hospital Doctors: Training for the Future.*[31]

2.13.2 Section 2.7 of our report has already touched on the way in which doctors in the Senior House Officer (SHO) grade fit into maternity care. In a woman centred service providers and professional bodies should be reviewing what value there is to pregnant women of having their antenatal consultation with inexperienced doctors at the beginning of their obstetric training, rather than with midwives.

2.13.3 Our view is that the role of the obstetric SHO needs to be re-examined. The emphasis needs to be much more on the training aspects of the job rather than the service commitments. This may mean that the number of trainees will need to be looked at in more detail.

2.13.4 This revised role will obviously have implications for midwives and the more senior grade doctors in obstetrics. Midwives will need to carry out some of those duties often undertaken by SHOs. If the training aspects of the SHOs' role are emphasised more strongly and their training programme becomes more structured then consultants will need to spend more time on teaching. There will need to be more consultants, but this is in line with the proposals set out in the Chief Medical Officer's working group report mentioned above. Experienced midwives, too, may become more formally involved in the training of SHOs and this is a factor which will need to be taken into account in their staffing levels.

2.13.5 If, as suggested in section 2.5, more antenatal care is to be in the community, then training should take place there, as well as in hospital. This will be of particular significance to trainee GPs, who will eventually be providing most of their care in the community.

---

[31] *Hospital Doctors: Training for the Future.* The report of the Working Group on specialist medical training. Department of Health. April 1993.

OBJECTIVE

The role and training of senior house officers working in obstetrics should be designed primarily to equip them with the skills and knowledge that they will require in order either to provide a full range of maternity services working as general practitioners, or to continue their education and training to become obstetricians.

ACTION POINTS

<u>Relevant professional bodies</u> should continue to review the education and training of obstetric senior house officers and make recommendations.

<u>Providers</u> should review working practices in their units to ensure that the duties undertaken by the SHO are appropriate to their needs and in line with the recommendations of the professional bodies.

3 Accessible Care

The Expert Group believes that the second principle underpinning woman centred care is that:

"Maternity services must be readily and easily accessible to all women. The should be sensitive to the needs of the local population and based primarily in the community."

The Expert Group was made increasingly aware that access to services was not easy for some women. Women who were assertive and articulate described the difficulties, and sometimes hostility, that they encountered when trying to establish which services were available to them. For women who were less confident, or those who found communication difficult, access to services was even more of a challenge.

3.1 Assessing local needs

3.1.1   During fact-finding visits to different parts of the country, we found that, although circumstances varied a great deal, in many places there was clear evidence of purchasers and providers being aware of local needs and tailoring services to suit those needs. In Scunthorpe, for example, midwifery services had been decentralised and small midwifery teams established providing care for women in discrete geographical areas. On some other visits, it seemed that services were designed to meet the needs of the professionals rather than those of the women.

3.1.2   The Group believes that local population profiles should be refined so that the purchaser can accurately assess the characteristics of the childbearing population. For example, the ethnic mix and the number of teenage, unsupported, homeless, or older mothers will need to be assessed. Purchasers should ensure that services specifications reflect any particular needs identified.

3.1.3   Through perinatal reviews and consumer satisfaction surveys, providers will also be able to identify women who have more complex needs than those usually encountered. Standards must then be agreed, and regular audit undertaken, to assess whether the needs of these women are being met effectively. It is important that the audit results are fed back to staff.

3.1.4   In their evidence, The Royal College of Midwives, the Royal College of Obstetricians and Gynaecologists, the National Childbirth Trust and the Maternity Alliance highlighted the importance of recognising the individual needs, wishes and views of all women. It is essential that the service is designed to be sensitive to their religious, cultural and linguistic needs. Staff training programmes should include these issues, but care must also be taken to emphasise the need to avoid stereotyping. A service that is responsive is more likely to be helpful and valued, and therefore more likely to be used.

3.1.5   Carol Baxter, a Health and Race Consultant, speaking at the Consensus Conference, highlighted how generalisations about particular groups can be unhelpful. She emphasised that variations between individuals within discrete ethnic and social groups may be as wide as those between the groups themselves. For example, there is a belief that the husbands of Asian women do not like to be present for the delivery of their child. While this may be true for some Asian men it is not true for all. We recommend that the preference of individuals should always be sought and respected.

OBJECTIVE

Services should be based on an understanding of local health, social and cultural needs.

ACTION POINTS

<u>**Purchasers**</u> **should involve consumers in assessing local needs and monitoring service delivery.**

<u>**Providers**</u> **should establish mechanisms for identifying women with more complex needs than are normally encountered.**

3.2 Lay representatives

3.2.1 The NHS Management Executive document *Local Voices*[32] is an excellent guide on how to involve those who would not normally put themselves forward as consumer representatives. It says, *"to give people an effective voice in the shaping of health services locally will call for a radically different approach from that employed in the past. In particular, there needs to be a move away from one-off consultation towards on-going involvement of local people in purchasing activities."*

3.2.2 It is becoming common practice for local National Childbirth Trust branches and Community Health Councils to have formal representation on bodies involved in planning maternity services. Such representation is warmly welcomed, and we hope it is a practice which will be adopted in areas where this is not yet happening.

3.2.3 Although Maternity Services Liaison Committees (MSLCs) were established in all the units that we visited, the membership of the groups varied considerably. We support the view of the Select Committee that MSLCs must be retained and their role strengthened. The MSLC, chaired by a lay person, should report primarily to the purchasers but will also need to refer to providers on local issues. Purchasers need to ensure that a MSLC is established within each purchasing authority and should also agree the committee's constitution and remit.

OBJECTIVE

Users of maternity services should be actively involved in planning and reviewing services. The lay representation must reflect the ethnic, cultural and social mix of the local population. A Maternity Services Liaison Committee should be established within every district health authority.

ACTION POINTS

<u>Purchasers</u> **should:**

* **ensure that effective Maternity Services Liaison Committees, with proper lay representation, including a lay chairperson, are established; and**

* **ensure that users of services, including those who do not normally take part in formal consumer groups, are actively involved in planning services.**

<u>Providers</u> **should ensure that users are actively involved in the planning, development and evaluation of services.**

---

[32]*Local Voices: the views of local people in purchasing for health*. Department of Health. 1992.

3.3 Communication and information

3.3.1   The problems resulting from poor communication were apparent to the Group in almost every aspect of the evidence we received. Women described the difficulties they sometimes encountered in trying to find out which services were available to them. Others set out very clearly the frustration they felt when trying to explain their wishes to staff who appeared at best disinterested, and at worst obstructive.

3.3.2   We acknowledged the professionals' view that they have an obligation to offer guidance, based on their professional knowledge, to women who are making choices about their maternity care. Unfortunately, what may be intended as guidance by the doctor or midwife may be seen as coercion by the woman concerned. Training in communication skills is essential for professionals and is dealt with in more detail in Section 3.7.

3.3.3   The *Survey of Good Communications Practice in Maternity Services* which forms Part II of this report outlines the key principles which should underpin the development of a communication strategy. The survey gives examples of innovative and dynamic initiatives from purchasers, providers, professional organisations, charities and voluntary groups and we commend it to the NHS. We hope it will be widely read and acted upon.

3.3.4   Communication strategies must pay careful attention to the availability of information. Women need to know what is available before they can begin to make choices about their care. Purchasers should publish information agreed by the health professionals involved about the range of services in their locality in an appropriate and accessible form. Providers too, need to make sure that women are informed in more detail about the different options available to them. It is important that written information material is widely available in family planning clinics, and women's health clinics; and, as recommended by the General Medical Services Committee, the Royal College of General Practitioners and the Royal College of Midwives[33], in other more readily accessible places such as post offices and libraries.

3.3.5   We support the view expressed by the Select Committee and endorsed by the Government in its response, that purchasers should publish annual figures relating to perinatal care. We recognise that there are practical difficulties in producing comparable data of this sort, but believe that every effort should be made to resolve these difficulties as soon as possible. We received evidence about the need to look at improving the completeness and quality of data collected through the maternity hospital episode system and linking it to birth registration data. Data collection systems will need to be developed in order to accommodate an increase in community-based services.

[33]See footnote to paragraph 2.2.3.

OBJECTIVE

Information about maternity services should be provided in a form appropriate and accessible to women.

ACTION POINTS

<u>The Department of Health</u> should:

*   develop a system of data collection which can be used locally and allows for meaningful comparison of statistics relating to perinatal care in both the community and the hospital;

<u>Purchasers and providers</u> should:

*   involve users in the development of information materials;

*   work together to improve the quality of data collected about the local population; and

*   where a need has been identified, make sure that information is provided in a form which can be used by those whose first language is not English.

3.4 Uptake of services

3.4.1 Almost all women receive some care during the antenatal period, but there is a wide variation both in the time that a woman first seeks care and the degree to which it is acceptable and appropriate to her needs.

3.4.2 The evidence we received, particularly from the Maternity Alliance and the National Childbirth Trust, showed that many women feel vulnerable when they are pregnant. This sense of vulnerability is likely to be heightened when the circumstances of the pregnancy are thought to be unusual or different in some way. This may make the woman reluctant to seek care.

3.4.3 For example, women who are very young when they become pregnant may fear feeling out of place or conspicuous in an antenatal clinic, and may therefore be reluctant to attend for care. It was apparent in some areas which we visited, particularly the more rural ones, that the woman's GP can be of great value, especially when the woman is known to him or her. In other areas, where populations are more transient, this is less likely to be the case.

3.4.4 Some providers are trying to make information about health services more readily available to young people. In Stockport the Group heard of a youth club which was used as a focus for health promotion activities and occasionally antenatal advice. This successful initiative gives young people the freedom to seek advice informally, and is to be welcomed as part of *The Health of the Nation* initiative to reduce the number of teenage pregnancies.

3.4.5 Speaking at the Consensus Conference, Margaret Anthony, Director of Women's Services at the Royal London Hospital Trust, described how a fundamental review of the needs of women living in Tower Hamlets had shown a particular need to adapt services for women who were recent immigrants from Sylhet in Bangladesh. The perinatal mortality rate had been higher in this group than in the indigenous population, and the women appeared to use services less often.

3.4.6 The managers of the service, initially liaising closely with women who were working in a community based, and independently funded, Maternity Services Liaison Scheme, developed a Women's Services Health Aides Scheme. This uses bilingual Sylheti-speaking health workers to work alongside and under the supervision of midwives. It has now been running for seven years, and is thought to have contributed to the reduction in the perinatal mortality rate among this group and to a much increased use of services.

3.4.7   Initiatives such as this, which draw on resources available in the community, attribute part of their success and acceptability to the early involvement of health workers who can most closely represent the particular group.

3.4.8   Some provider units will find that they are caring for women whose particular needs make them more than usually vulnerable, for example women who are misusing drugs, or who have been diagnosed as being HIV positive or having AIDS. It is essential that the needs of these women are identified early and that they are made to feel welcome and wanted by the professionals providing care. Women in these situations can be very wary of professionals who, they fear, may be making judgements about their lifestyles or those of their partners.

3.4.9   When a unit is providing care on a regular basis for women with such problems, providers should consider establishing a small team which could offer the particular support and expertise required. Cooperation between the different professions is essential in these circumstances. At Saint Mary's Hospital in Paddington, one midwife offers additional care and support to women who are HIV positive. This has proved beneficial to the women, and has allowed the midwife to develop a high level of knowledge and skill while working in close liaison with experts in this field.

3.4.10   We were impressed with some innovative initiatives aimed at addressing the particular needs of some women. For example, in Bloomsbury and Islington, the work of community midwives took special account of the large population of homeless mothers. Information was posted in local bed and breakfast accommodation about services which were available to women at the local health centre, including details of community midwife clinics and advice about self-referral. In another, more rural, area a midwife had established a very strong rapport with a group of travellers. Both of these approaches to care gave the women a firm and accessible link with the service. We commend such initiatives.

3.4.11   The MORI survey showed that 2 women in 100 were not registered with a general practitioner when they had their last baby. The Group is aware that, in some instances, women in this situation have found it difficult to obtain maternity care without a letter of referral from a general practitioner. We also recognise that the women most likely to find themselves in this situation are women who are homeless, refugees or travellers. We urge purchasers and providers to take measures to ensure that the service does not discriminate against these women. It should positively encourage them to seek care with a professional of their choice and advise them how they and their family may register with a GP if they wish to do so.

3.4.12   Where purchasers and providers identify areas of particular need, a strategy to meet the need should be designed and agreed. The importance of involving consumers, lay organisations and appropriate specialists in the development of the strategy cannot be overemphasised.

OBJECTIVE

Regular monitoring of the uptake of services should take place in order to identify those women who are least likely to seek care and use the service to their full advantage. A strategy should then be developed to ensure that services are accessible to those women.

ACTION POINTS

<u>Purchasers and providers</u> should:

*   agree ways of monitoring the use of services and their effectiveness for women with different needs; and

*   develop a strategy to ensure that services are readily accessible to these women including those who are not registered with a GP.

3.5 Women with disabilities

3.5.1   It is important that services reflect the needs of women who have disabilities and ensure that action is taken to overcome the obstacles which confront them. While physical obstructions are of course a frustrating problem, there are other equally daunting barriers resulting from the prejudice and ignorance of able-bodied professionals.

3.5.2   Providers must ensure that the needs of people with disabilities are recognised and incorporated into the planning and provision of maternity services. There should be collaboration with consumer organisations from the earliest stages. The Group acknowledges the pioneering role of the Maternity Alliance, working with women with disabilities, in attempting to present a comprehensive picture of the full range of their needs.

3.5.3   Some women will have disabilities, possibly with underlying medical problems, which are encountered rarely by midwives and obstetricians. These professionals should acknowledge that the woman will probably be the best source of information about her condition, but they should also seek help and advice from colleagues and others with appropriate expertise. Voluntary organisations can also be a useful source of advice to professionals, and perhaps more importantly, to the woman herself.

3.5.4   The particular challenges some women with disabilities may face often only become apparent to professionals when women present for care. Care should be planned jointly with the woman and any appropriate specialists according to her individual needs and wishes, in the same way as for other pregnant women.

3.5.5   In information gathered by the Maternity Alliance, of 87 women responding to a general question, almost half (46%) used the opportunity to comment on the apparent lack of training of staff in this area. A woman who was deaf described how the only way one midwife felt able to communicate with her was by giving her a very definite "thumbs-up" sign each time she passed her in the corridor.

3.5.6   Deaf parents may be made to feel isolated if maternity care is inappropriate to their needs. In Manchester [34], the Maternity Care for the Deaf Project has been running for four years. By developing an increased understanding of "deaf awareness" and the various communication methods employed by deaf people through study days, workshops and a book produced by staff at the Wythenshaw Maternity Hospital, Manchester, midwives have been enabled to adapt maternity care specifically for the deaf.

[34] *Maternity care for the Deaf.* Jennifer Kelsall et al. Further details are given in *Changing Childbirth Part II: Survey of Good Communications Practice in Maternity Services*

3.5.7 Initiatives like this give parents with disabilities better access to information, and enable them to make informed choices antenatally, in labour and postnatally.

OBJECTIVE

Women with disabilities should have full access to services and have confidence that their needs are fully understood.

ACTION POINTS

<u>Purchasers</u> should ensure that service specifications incorporate the needs of women with disabilities.

<u>Providers</u> should design and modify facilities to make them accessible to women with disabilities.

3.6 Making best use of the services

3.6.1 The issue of access to maternity services is not just about a woman's first contact with them. It was apparent that many women attended regularly for every appointment and had many interactions with professionals, but never really felt they were involved in the decisions about their care.

3.6.2 Providers must ensure that the woman is seen as the focus of care and that her views and needs are respected. When women have more complex needs, or if they find it difficult to articulate them, care must be taken to create a genuine opportunity for the woman to explain her views and concerns. The move towards a community based system of antenatal care, as we saw in Scunthorpe and Medway, had discernible strengths. Here, care usually took place in the woman's home, where she was more likely to feel relaxed and unhurried, and therefore more able to express her worries.

3.6.3 When a maternity unit is providing services to significant numbers of women who are unable to communicate in English, it is essential that providers should develop link worker and advocacy schemes. Women who do not speak English must be given the means of expressing their wishes and exercising choice. They should be kept fully informed of all matters relevant to their care. Link workers and advocates should not be seen as optional extras to the service. They should be fully integrated into the maternity care team, with clearly defined roles, appropriate training and education opportunities.

3.6.4 Strategies to increase uptake of services should be designed to attract a wide range of people. Images of women, children and families from a wide spectrum of backgrounds, including those with disabilities, should be used in health promotion material. The tendency to use photographs of black women only when dealing with ethnic issues, and pictures of women with disabilities only when wishing to identify them as different, has the effect of marginalising them and should be avoided.

3.6.5 We think that it is essential for purchasers, working in close liaison with consumers, to monitor the services regularly and to assess whether they are equally accessible to all women. Purchasers must ensure that audit of consumers' experiences of the service takes place on a regular basis. This subject is explored more fully in Chapter 4.

OBJECTIVE

All women should have the opportunity to be fully involved in their care.

ACTION POINTS

<u>Providers</u> should establish ways, including link worker and advocacy schemes, of supporting women whose first language is not English to enable them to participate fully in their care.

3.7 Education and training

3.7.1 Staff education and training is a key element in meeting the diversity of women's needs. It is part of the provider's role to ensure that staff are able to take advantage of training opportunities which will help them to help women. With the growing awareness of the need for effective medical audit we hope that increasingly joint clinical audit and training will be introduced.

3.7.2 Communications skills are particularly important. The provision of clear and unbiased information enables a woman to make informed choices and take an active part in decisions about her care. The Group recognises that presenting information about maternity care in this way is not easy. Medical and midwifery education does already include an element of communication skills training, but we recommend that existing staff should be able to improve their skills as part of their on-going education.

3.7.3 Part II of this report details a two-year research project on this subject, completed in June 1993, at the United Medical and Dental Schools of Guy's and St Thomas' Hospitals. Funded by the Medical Research Council, it has focused on communication problems in antenatal clinics, and the design of training programmes for health professionals to improve their communication skills. The results showed that training led to more information being given to women and some improvement in the overall knowledge of antenatal tests.

3.7.4 In areas where there are significant numbers of women from different ethnic groups, it is important for staff to be aware of the cultural and religious beliefs which influence lifestyles and should therefore influence care. Education should help staff to be sensitive, non-patronising and, above all, sympathetic and kind. This will be of great benefit to the women involved but it will also help staff. They will have more confidence in their own abilities to deal successfully with situations which might previously have appeared unfamiliar and therefore intimidating.

3.7.5 We recognise that this is a complex area. On-going education and training must be available to ensure that staff are knowledgeable, and that they have the skills to give appropriate care in these circumstances.

OBJECTIVE

Staff should have received training to enable them to support all women with different needs so that they can use the service to maximum advantage.

ACTION POINTS

<u>Providers, statutory and professional bodies</u> should ensure that all staff have access to training which is designed to help them understand the differing needs women may have.

4 *Effective and Efficient Services*

The Expert Group believes that the third principle underpinning the provision of maternity services is that

"Women should be involved in the monitoring and planning of maternity services to ensure that they are responsive to the needs of a changing society. In addition the service should be effective and resources used efficiently."

Tradition plays a large part in the way maternity care is provided. The Group saw a good deal of evidence that practice was not always based on measures known to be effective. In spite of the recommendations presented in Effective Care in Pregnancy and Childbirth[35], which are now continuously updated in The Cochrane Collaboration Pregnancy and Childbirth Database, ineffective and unproven practices continue.

Purchasers have a key role in ensuring that providers implement practices of proven benefit and abandon those which have been demonstrated as ineffective. When the effect or benefit of a practice is unclear, it should be systematically evaluated. Existing patterns of practice and organisation of services should not be exempt from evaluation.

4.1 Strategic plans

4.1.1   There are already some impressive local initiatives to improve maternity services. However, in many areas change is still essential if the service is to become properly focused on women's needs. This change must be managed, and purchasers must take overall responsibility for making sure that it is made in a structured and orderly way.

4.1.2   For purchasers, a key step in this process will be to draw up a comprehensive long term strategy for maternity services in their area. They need to look forward over a five year period, and develop a strategy with clear aims, service targets and milestones on the way to meeting them. This will allow providers to plan and manage changes to their services which can meet the aims specified by purchasers. It will also help to provide stability and continuity in a framework of change.

4.1.3   The basic principles of a strategy for maternity care will be no different to those applied to other areas of purchasing health services. It should contain clear health targets and identify how progress towards them will be measured.

[35]*Effective Care in Pregnancy and Childbirth.* Chalmers, Enkin and Keirse. Oxford University Press. 1989.

4.1.4   Women live in communities, and not in hospitals. This report has already stressed that to improve quality the maternity services must be more oriented to women and their needs. Services, especially antenatal care, should in general be located more accessibly taking into account factors such as public transport. A key feature of local strategies must therefore be to make services more community-based. This shift should be monitored to maximise the speed with which changes take place while minimising any short term disruption.

OBJECTIVE

Within a period of 5 years providers should be able to demonstrate a significant shift towards a more community-oriented service.

ACTION POINTS

Purchasers must develop strategic plans for maternity services, with guidance on future purchasing intentions showing positive moves towards woman centred and community-based care.

4.2 Monitoring contracts

4.2.1   It is vital that women are involved in the planning and shaping of services. Purchasers should continue to improve and develop information systems to assess overall needs and produce detailed profiles for use as the foundation of their planning. But this is not a substitute for listening to women's views about the care they would like to receive and acting upon the information that they give.

4.2.2   Monitoring contracts is an important purchaser function. To give increased choice and control to women, the views of users of the service should be an important element of monitoring. Women and their families should be asked to contribute by taking part in consumer surveys, and by helping design methods of getting feedback from people who use the services. Formal channels such as Community Health Councils and Maternity Services Liaison Committees can also provide significant input. But purchasers must seek ways of reaching those who are not normally involved in these types of organisation.

4.2.3   Initiatives such as the Priority Search used by North Derbyshire Health Authority are one way of securing feedback from women who use the services. This technique identifies the key values which underlie the preferences of users for different types of maternity care. For example, women might be asked to assign relative priorities to issues such as local access, continuity of carer, availability of specialist services and so on.

4.2.4   Another way is through consumer surveys. In 1989 the Department of Health issued to all health authorities a standard pack, produced by the Office of Population, Censuses and Surveys[36], to assist them in carrying out consumer surveys. The Group recommends the continued use of this pack.

[36] *Women's experience of maternity care – a survey manual:* Office of Population, Censuses and Surveys. HMSO 1989; and *Getting Consumers' Views of Maternity Care;* Jo Garcia, NPEU. Department of Health 1989.

OBJECTIVE

The views of women who use the service should be regularly monitored and services adjusted to reflect their needs.

ACTION POINTS

<u>Purchasers and Providers</u> should agree a monitoring system to enable them to achieve this objective.

4.3 Research and audit

4.3.1   There is a long history in maternity services of well-intentioned changes which are not backed-up with proper research-based evidence to support their introduction. The widespread use of continuous electronic fetal monitoring has already been mentioned in Chapter 2. This is just one example of the way in which technological developments have been adopted as common practice, without distinguishing whether they are really necessary or beneficial. This is also true for other techniques and practices such as water birth, homeopathy and aromatherapy. The Group heard evidence from Iain Chalmers (Director of the Cochrane Centre) and others which highlighted the need for new practices to be tested formally. Where women express a wish for a particular form of care which has no proven benefit, this fact must be discussed with them openly and fairly.

4.3.2   The other side of this coin is that in some cases where there is sound evidence about particular techniques or practices, it is not always applied. One example presented to the Group was that of research published in 1989 by Grant et al[37] suggesting that the use of glycerol-impregnated catgut to repair perineal trauma can result in increased pain and discomfort during intercourse for up to three years following delivery. Despite the evidence, use of glycerol-impregnated catgut continued in some maternity units.

4.3.3   Another example is the well published work about the value of cortico-steroids administered antenatally where a preterm birth is anticipated[38]. The success of this practice in reducing Respiratory Distress Syndrome and mortality in babies has been demonstrated. Its cost-effectiveness has been acknowledged and the work has been widely disseminated throughout the NHS, but it has not been acted upon universally.

4.3.4   We were encouraged by the fact that there is now much greater emphasis on research into maternity care practice. In a service which aims to provide the best for women and their babies the benefits and hazards of techniques used must be rigorously assessed. The Group also supported the views about the value of audit expressed in much of the evidence received. In particular, we welcomed the fact that the General Medical Services Committee, the Royal College of General Practitioners and the Royal College of Midwives had included a list of suggested criteria for joint clinical audit in maternity care in their evidence to the Group[39].

[37]Grant A, Sleep J, Ashurst H, Spencer JAD. *Dyspareunia associated with the use of glycerol-impregnated catgut to repair perineal trauma - report of a three-year follow-up study.* Br J Obstet Gynaecol 1989; Vol 96: pp741-3

[38]*Effective Care in Pregnancy and Childbirth.* Chalmers, Enkin and Kierse. Oxford University Press 1989. Volume 1 Chapter 45: Promoting pulmonary maturity.

[39]See footnote to paragraph 2.2.3

OBJECTIVE

Clinical practice should be based on sound evidence and be subject to regular clinical audit.

ACTION POINTS

<u>Purchasers</u> should agree with providers quality standards based on current evidence of effectiveness of treatment and procedures.

<u>Providers</u> should review their procedures for clinical audit.

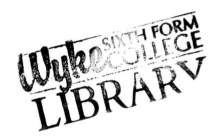

4.4 Evaluation of new patterns of care

4.4.1   Organisational changes to the provision of care should also be evaluated. The IMS study of team midwifery mentioned in paragraph 2.3.7 noted that in many places where a "team scheme" had been introduced, there had been no systematic evaluation of the new arrangements. Where significant changes are introduced, evaluation is vital. Clear goals should be set and basic audit used to check whether these are being met. The importance of asking women using the service for their views cannot be stressed enough.

4.4.2   There are a number of sources of expert advice which can be called upon when devising an evaluation methodology. The National Perinatal Epidemiology Unit in Oxford, the Institute of Epidemiology and Health Services Research at the University of Leeds and the Royal College of Obstetricians and Gynaecologists' Audit Unit in Manchester, are all excellent resources. Wherever possible the results of evaluations should be published so that others may share the evidence collected.

OBJECTIVES

New patterns of service should be designed to allow evaluation of both their effectiveness and their acceptability to women using the service.

ACTION POINTS

<u>Purchasers</u> should agree with providers the objectives of new approaches to providing health care and the methods for evaluating them.

4.5 Use of resources

4.5.1 The Group recognised that effective services tend to be efficient services. In this respect the maternity service is no different from any other area of the NHS. Purchasers must look for ways to maximise efficiency in the use of the resources available to them for the benefit of women. The Select Committee heard from users and professionals alike, of their concern about the duplication which takes place in maternity care.

4.5.2 This duplication of effort benefits no-one. For individual women, there is the cost of time wasted in appointments with different professionals who ask the same questions or carry out the same procedures. On a wider scale, there is the financial cost of employing different professionals who go over the same ground time and time again.

4.5.3 The appropriate use of the skills of different professionals was another matter raised both with the Select Committee and the Expert Group. The training of midwives equips them to care for women with uncomplicated pregnancies. The resources tied up in consultants seeing these same women, if the women themselves do not seek consultant involvement, needs to be reviewed. These are issues which purchasers should investigate with providers and possibly family health services authorities during their reviews of maternity care.

4.5.4 This report has already set out our concerns about the effectiveness of two aspects of antenatal care – the package of antenatal care offered to women with uncomplicated pregnancies, and the increasing introduction of antenatal day assessment units. The issue of efficient use of resources arises in both these areas. If the recommended changes to the provision of antenatal care were to be made, the health service should be able to use more effectively the resources at present locked into this particular pattern of care.

4.5.5 The use of antenatal day assessment units is said to bring down antenatal admissions to hospital, and yet there does not appear to be a consequent reduction of any significance. In areas such as this, with high capital costs, purchasers must ask providers to justify this spending with evidence of potential improvement. We recommend that the Central Research and Development Committee's Standing Group on Health Technology should look at this area.

OBJECTIVE

The service provided must represent value for money and the cost and benefits of alternative arrangements assessed locally.

ACTION POINTS

<u>Purchasers</u> should agree with providers a programme to review the use of current resources, with particular emphasis on reducing unnecessary duplication.

5 *Action for Change*

5.1 Introduction

5.1.1   This report has identified the three key principles which we believe must underlie effective woman centred maternity services. The objectives which will fulfil those principles and the action needed to meet them are summarised at Annex 1.

5.1.2   Meeting these objectives will require action on a broad front. It will mean changes to service organisation, education and training, the role of different professions and the planning and monitoring of services. Most of all, it will require a recognition of the central role of the woman in planning the care for her baby and for herself.

5.2 Action

5.2.1   Many different groups will have a part to play. *Purchasers* will need to review the services available to their local population, and draw up strategic plans. They should take into account all the objectives set out in this report in a way that is sensitive to the social, cultural and ethnic characteristics of the community. They should then agree targets with provider units in moving towards services that are more woman centred and community-oriented. *Consumers* should be fully involved in the planning of services, drawing up specifications, quality standards and monitoring.

5.2.2   *Providers* will need to review their philosophies for care, their current practices and their organisation to assess how well they meet the key principles. They should design services so that they meet the differing individual needs of all women. In particular, they should review the role and organisation of midwives and identify how far the criteria for continuity of carer are being met.

5.2.3   Both *purchasers and providers* should provide clear information for users about the services available to them, and the standards they should expect. They should take a much more critical approach to the effectiveness of different practices and techniques.

5.2.4   *Clinicians* will need to agree clinical guidelines and develop effective teamwork across the different professional groups. *Professional and statutory bodies* will need to continue to develop education and training to meet the needs of the future service. *Consumer groups* should play an active role in assessing services on behalf of the women using them, and work with purchasers and providers to bring about change.

5.3 Indicators of success

5.3.1 Purchasers and providers will need to agree in their strategic plans and contracts a range of goals and standards to be achieved and the way in which progress can be monitored. The Group identified ten key indicators of success. If these are achieved, much of what we have recommended will have been put into place.

INDICATORS OF SUCCESS

Within 5 years

1. All women should be entitled to carry their own notes.

2. Every woman should know one midwife who ensures continuity of her midwifery care – the named midwife.

3. At least 30% of women should have the midwife as the lead professional.

4. Every woman should know the lead professional who has a key role in the planning and provision of her care.

5. At least 75% of women should know the person who cares for them during their delivery.

6. Midwives should have direct access to some beds in all maternity units.

7. At least 30% of women delivered in a maternity unit should be admitted under the management of the midwife.

8. The total number of antenatal visits for women with uncomplicated pregnancies should have been reviewed in the light of the available evidence and the RCOG guidelines.

9. All front line ambulances should have a paramedic able to support the midwife who needs to transfer a woman to hospital in an emergency.

10. All women should have access to information about the services available in their locality.

5.3.2   We do not underestimate the hard work and commitment that will be needed to reach these goals. However, while on visits and in reviewing the evidence that we received we were frequently impressed by the skill, dedication and compassion of the people working in maternity services. From the progress seen in services in different parts of the country, we consider that these are realistic targets to be achieved nationally within 5 years.

5.3.3   The first step at the local level is for all purchasers to review their services and draw up a strategic plan during 1994/95. Initial targets for change should be introduced by 1995/96. Providers should review their current organisation and practices. At national level a short-term taskforce will be set up to monitor progress, encourage demonstration sites and innovation, and share good practice. This taskforce will report to the NHS Management Executive who will provide Ministers with regular updates on progress.

5.4 Conclusion

5.4.1   This report is a manifesto for change in the way maternity services are planned and provided. There are some who may find its proposals surprising, but many others who see much familiar in its pages. There is a wealth of good practice up and down the country on which we can build.

5.4.2   The Expert Group has been impressed by the kindness in the service, and the genuine desire on the part of health professionals and managers to help women remain well and give birth to healthy babies. Sometimes, however, their efforts have been frustrated by an inflexible and traditional system of care which is ill-designed to meet individual needs and preferences.

5.4.3   Change is never easy. There will, naturally, be some who oppose it. We sincerely hope, however, that their reluctance and their fears will be overcome by proof that the new methods not only work but provide increased satisfaction, not only for the women and their families using the service, but also for those working within it.

5.4.4   The Group believes there is a new spirit abroad in maternity services which can be harnessed to bring about change. Our greatest hope is that, in five years' time, the principles embodied in this report will have become so widely accepted and its practices so commonplace that *Changing Childbirth* will have done its work and can take its place on the shelf of history.

Glossary

ACCESSIBLE CARE: Care which women are able to reach and to receive.

ADVOCATE: A person who takes up issues about the care of a pregnant woman on her behalf and challenges practices in the NHS to meet her needs. An advocate is usually able to communicate with the pregnant woman in her own language.

ANTENATAL CARE: Care of women during pregnancy by doctors and midwives in order to predict and detect problems with the mother or the unborn child. Advice is also offered on other matters relevant to pregnancy and birth.

AUDIT: The *evaluation* of care against a standard, with the purpose of improving practice, where necessary, within the audited group. (See also *clinical audit* and *medical audit*.)

BAG AND MASK RESUSCITATION: Manual revival using an air-refillable bag and close fitting face mask to push air into the lungs.

BIRTH PLAN: A written record of a woman's preferences for her care and that of her unborn child during labour and childbirth.

CAESARIAN SECTION: An operation by which the baby is delivered through an incision in the abdominal wall and uterus.

CLINICAL AUDIT: The assessment by groups of *professionals* of care they have provided against a standard, with the purpose of improving practice, where necessary, within the audited group. (See also *audit* and *medical audit*.)

COMPLICATED PREGNANCY: A pregnancy in which a risk of complication is evident *or* in which a complication occurs.

CONSUMER: A *user* of the maternity services; the pregnant woman.

DOMINO: Abbreviation of "domiciliary in/out". This is a model of maternity care in which women are taken into hospital in labour by their own midwife who delivers them and then transfers them home shortly after birth.

DOWN'S SYNDROME: A chromosomal problem which causes a baby to be born with severe learning difficulties.

EFFECTIVE: Proven to achieve an objective.

EFFICIENT: Achieves an objective economically.

EPIDURAL ANAESTHESIA: A local anaesthetic injected around the spinal sac causing complete loss of sensation in the lower part of the body, to a level which allows a surgical procedure to be undertaken in that area without pain.

EPIDURAL ANALGESIA: A local anaesthetic injected around the spinal sac causing some numbness in the lower part of the body. It relieves labour pains effectively.

EVALUATION: Assessment of the relative merits of a procedure or pattern of care.

FETAL: Of *fetus.*

FETUS: The unborn child.

HEALTH DISTRICT: A defined geographical area, within which health care services are purchased for the resident population by a district health authority or agent acting on behalf of the authority (see *purchaser*).

INTERVENTION: Clinical procedure in pregnancy or labour, for example induction of labour or delivery of a baby with the aid of instruments, or by *caesarian section.*

INTRAPARTUM: During labour.

INTUBATION: The passing of a tube into the trachea to establish an unobstructed airway.

LEAD PROFESSIONAL: The professional who will give a substantial part of the care personally *and* who is responsible for ensuring that the woman has access to care from other professionals, as appropriate.

LINKWORKER: A person who acts as an advisor on healthcare issues, and in some cases will also provide interpreting services. A linkworker will be able to communicate with the pregnant woman in her own language.

MATERNITY HOSPITAL EPISODE SYSTEM: A system of collecting statistics about the level and distribution of activity in the NHS maternity services. The statistics are collected by the Office of Population, Censuses and Surveys on behalf of the Department of Health.

MATERNITY SERVICES LIAISON COMMITTEE: A local committee which brings together all the professions involved in maternity care with lay representatives of the women who use the services, with the purpose of agreeing procedures and monitoring their effectiveness as they apply to women. MSLCs were first defined in the report of the Maternity Services Advisory Committee (see footnote to Introduction, paragraph 2).

MATERNITY UNIT: A building or group of buildings in which maternity care is provided. It can be located within or adjacent to a general hospital, or away from the general hospital.

MEDICAL AUDIT: The assessment by doctors of medical care they have provided against a standard, with the purpose of improving practice, where necessary, within the audited group. (See also *audit* and *clinical audit*.)

MIDWIFE/GP UNIT: A *maternity unit* in which midwives and/or general practitioners are the professionals leading the maternity care.

NAMED MIDWIFE: It is a Patient's Charter Standard that a woman should have a named, qualified midwife who will be responsible for her midwifery care.

NEONATAL: The first 28 days of life in a baby.

OBSTETRIC FLYING SQUAD: A specialist team providing an emergency obstetric service outside hospital.

PERINATAL: The time of birth and the first week of life.

PERINATAL MORTALITY RATE: The number of *stillbirths* plus deaths in the first week of life per thousand total births.

PHARMACOLOGICAL PAIN RELIEF: The relief of pain through the administration of drugs.

PHYSIOLOGICAL: In accordance with the natural functions of the body.

POPULATION PROFILE: The description of a population group which takes particular account of the characteristics of the people within it, such as age mix, general state of health, ethnic and social mix.

PRENATAL: During pregnancy; antenatal.

PROFESSIONAL: In the context of this report, *professional* usually refers to the general practitioner, the midwife and/or the obstetrician, but includes anaesthetists, paediatricians and other specialists as appropriate.

PROVIDER: A hospital, NHS trust or unit providing maternity services.

PRIMIGRAVIDAE: Women who are pregnant for the first time.

PUERPERIUM: The 6 weeks immediately following childbirth.

PURCHASER: A health authority, or agent acting on behalf of the authority, to purchase health services for a local population.

POSTNATAL: Pertaining to the few weeks following birth.

RESPIRATORY DISTRESS SYNDROME: A lung disorder which results in difficulty with breathing. It occurs in some babies born several weeks before term.

STILLBIRTH: A baby born dead after 24 completed weeks gestation.

USER: A *consumer* of the maternity services; the pregnant woman.

Annex 1

SUMMARY OF ACTION POINTS

CHAPTER 2

Section 2.2

OBJECTIVE

Women should be fully involved when decisions are to be made about their care. They should have a choice regarding the professional who will lead their care and should, if they wish, carry their own case notes. They should be kept fully informed on matters relating to their care.

ACTION POINTS

<u>Purchasers</u> should:

*   ensure that providers are achieving these objectives through the contracting and monitoring process.

<u>Providers</u> should:

*   ensure that the services of a midwife are readily accessible to women when they first seek care;

*   make the necessary arrangements to ensure that all women are able to carry their case notes if they wish; and

*   ensure that women are fully informed on matters relating to their care and are fully involved when decisions are to be made about their care.

Section 2.3

OBJECTIVE

Every woman should have the name of a midwife who works locally, is known to her and whom she can contact for advice. She should also know the name of the lead professional who is responsible for planning and monitoring her care. Within 5 years, 75% of women should be cared for in labour by a midwife whom they have come to know during pregnancy.

ACTION POINTS

<u>Purchasers and providers</u> should develop a strategy which ensures that:

*   the named midwife and lead professional concepts are fully implemented within an agreed time scale; and

*   progress towards these objectives is carefully monitored.

Section 2.4

OBJECTIVE

A woman with an uncomplicated pregnancy should, if she wishes, be able to book with a midwife as the lead professional for the entire episode of care including delivery in a general hospital.

ACTION POINTS

<u>Purchasers</u> should:

*   ensure through their service specifications that women can book with a midwife for their entire episode of care; and

*   ensure that all women who become pregnant are informed about this option.

<u>Providers</u> should

*   ensure appropriate arrangements are in place to enable a woman to book with a midwife as her lead professional for her entire episode of care, including delivery in hospital.

Section 2.5

OBJECTIVE

Antenatal care should be provided so as to maximise the use of resources. It should also ensure that the woman and her partner feel supported and fully informed throughout the pregnancy, and are prepared for the birth and the care of their baby.

ACTION POINTS

<u>Purchasers</u> should:

*   agree a timetable for a review of antenatal care with the providers and monitor whether that timetable is being achieved.

<u>Providers</u> should:

* review the pattern of antenatal care in the light of current evidence;

* where they exist, establish clear objectives for antenatal assessment units and evaluate whether these objectives are being achieved;

* undertake a full review of parent-education sessions and if necessary develop a strategy for change; and

* review the counselling arrangements for prenatal screening tests.

Section 2.6

OBJECTIVE

Women should receive clear, unbiased advice and be able to choose where they would like their baby to be born. Their right to make that choice should be respected and every practical effort made to achieve the outcome that the woman believes is best for her baby and herself.

ACTION POINTS

<u>Purchasers</u> should:

* as part of their strategic plan, review the current choices available to women regarding the place of birth. Following consultation, these should be developed as appropriate for their locality and ensure that home birth is a real option for the women who may wish to have it; and

* ensure that women receive information about the full range of options for place of birth available in their locality.

<u>Providers</u> should:

* review their current organisation and practices to ensure that real choice about the place of birth is available; and

* develop a flexible system of care so that women are able to take time in making their decision regarding the place of birth, and can alter that decision close to the time of birth if they so wish.

Section 2.7

OBJECTIVE

When emergency services are required by the woman or her baby at, or around, the time of birth, they should be of the highest standard that can be achieved in the circumstances.

ACTION POINTS

<u>Purchasers</u> should:

*   agree a timetable with ambulance services for the target of one paramedic on each frontline ambulance able to offer appropriate support to the midwife in caring for the woman in an emergency.

<u>Providers</u> should:

*   review procedures for dealing with emergencies, including lines of communication;

*   establish a formal on-going staff training and updating programme dealing with common neonatal emergency procedures taking account of the guidance available in the British Paediatric Association Working Party Report on Neonatal Resuscitation; and

*   ensure that consultant obstetricians are prepared to offer advice and as much support as is practicable to midwives undertaking home births. This is in addition to the support already provided by the local supervisor of midwives.

Section 2.8

OBJECTIVE

Women should have the opportunity to discuss their plans for labour and birth. Their decisions should be recorded in their birth plans and this should be incorporated into their case notes. Every reasonable effort should be made to accommodate the wishes of the woman and her partner, and to inform them of the services that are available to them.

ACTION POINTS

<u>Purchasers</u> should:

*   use service specifications to ensure that the care of a woman in labour is flexible and able to accommodate the woman's individual needs and preferences; and

*   assess whether the objective is being achieved by auditing consumer satisfaction.

<u>Providers</u> should:

*   ensure that women have the opportunity to explore and discuss their wishes regarding labour and birth with a midwife or obstetrician;

*   ensure that the woman's wishes are recorded in her birth plan; and

*   have agreed guidelines for the care of women in labour which include
        guidance on obtaining anaesthetic and paediatric advice.

Section 2.9

OBJECTIVE

A woman who gives birth in hospital should return home, as far as is practicable, when she feels ready. Once home, she should be supported by her midwife, knowing that the general practitioner is available if medical advice is necessary. The pattern of support should be appropriate to the woman's needs and planned in consultation with her.

ACTION POINTS

<u>Providers</u> should:

*   have as flexible an approach as is practicable to the length of postnatal stay.
        This should normally be decided by the mother, following consultation with
        the midwife and obstetrician if appropriate;

*   have a flexible approach to postnatal home visiting ensuring that the views of
        the woman and her family determine the level of support provided by the
        midwife and health visitor;

*   monitor patterns of infant feeding and assess whether women are receiving
        appropriate information and advice, and feel confident with the method they
        have chosen; and

*   ensure that advice from a consultant paediatrician is available to a midwife
        working in the community should it be required.

Section 2.10

OBJECTIVE

GPs who wish to provide maternity care should receive appropriate training and encouragement to do so. Midwives and GPs should work in partnership in the best interests of the woman.

ACTION POINTS

<u>Professional and training bodies</u> should:

*   continue the development and implementation of appropriate training for
        GPs.

<u>Department of Health</u> should:

* consider with other Health Departments the need to review with the profession the current fee structure to encourage those GPs who wish to contribute substantially to maternity care; and

* consider with other Health Departments the need to review with the profession the criteria for the inclusion of GPs on the obstetric list.

Section 2.11

OBJECTIVE

The part which the midwife plays in maternity care should make full use of all her skills and knowledge, and reflect the full role for which she has been trained.

ACTION POINTS

<u>Purchasers and providers</u> should:

* ensure that midwives' skills are fully used by developing schemes that achieve continuity of carer; and

* ensure that there are appropriate updating programmes for midwives who are moving into new areas of practice.

Section 2.12

OBJECTIVE

The knowledge and skill of the obstetrician should be used primarily to provide advice, support and expertise for those women who have complicated pregnancies.

ACTION POINTS

<u>Purchasers and providers</u> should:

* agree a strategy with obstetricians and midwives to ensure that this objective is achieved;

* ensure that women with uncomplicated pregnancies are given the opportunity to meet a consultant obstetrician; and

* ensure that women with uncomplicated pregnancies can choose to book with a consultant obstetrician as their lead professional, via their GP or midwife.

Section 2.13

OBJECTIVE

The role and training of senior house officers working in obstetrics should be designed primarily to equip them with the skills and knowledge that they will require in order either to provide a full range of maternity services working as general practitioners, or to continue their education and training to become obstetricians.

ACTION POINTS

<u>Relevant professional bodies</u> should

*   continue to review the education and training of obstetric senior house officers and make recommendations.

<u>Providers</u> should:

*   review working practices in their units to ensure that the duties undertaken by the SHO are appropriate to their needs and in line with the recommendations of the professional bodies.

CHAPTER 3

Section 3.1

OBJECTIVE

Services should be based on an understanding of local health, social and cultural needs.

ACTION POINTS

<u>Purchasers</u> should:

*   involve consumers in assessing local needs and monitoring service delivery.

<u>Providers</u> should:

*   establish mechanisms for identifying women with more complex needs than are normally encountered.

Section 3.2

OBJECTIVE

Users of maternity services should be actively involved in planning and reviewing services. The lay representation must reflect the ethnic, cultural and social mix of the local population. A Maternity Services Liaison Committee should be established within every district health authority.

ACTION POINTS

<u>Purchasers</u> should:

*   ensure that effective Maternity Services Liaison Committees, with proper lay representation, including a lay chairperson, are established; and

*   ensure that users of services, including those who do not normally take part in formal consumer groups, are actively involved in planning services.

<u>Providers</u> should:

*   ensure that users are actively involved in the planning, development and evaluation of services.

Section 3.3

OBJECTIVE

Information about local maternity services should be provided in a form appropriate and accessible to women.

ACTION POINTS

The Department of Health should:

*   develop a system of data collection which can be used locally and allows for meaningful comparison of statistics relating to perinatal care in both the community and the hospital;

Purchasers and providers should:

*   involve users in the development of information materials;

*   work together to improve the quality of data collected about the local population; and

*   where a need has been identified, make sure that information is provided in a form which can be used by those whose first language is not English.

Section 3.4

OBJECTIVE

Regular monitoring of the uptake of services should take place in order to identify those women who are least likely to seek care and use the service to their full advantage. A strategy should then be developed to ensure that services are accessible to those women.

ACTION POINTS

Purchasers and providers should:

*   agree ways of monitoring the use of services and their effectiveness for women with different needs; and

*   develop a strategy to ensure that services are readily accessible to these women, including those who are not registered with a GP.

Section 3.5

OBJECTIVE

Women with disabilities should have full access to services and have confidence that their needs are fully understood.

ACTION POINTS

<u>Purchasers</u> should:

*   ensure that service specifications incorporate the needs of women with disabilities.

<u>Providers</u> should:

*   design and modify facilities to make them accessible to women with disabilities.

Section 3.6

OBJECTIVE

All women should have the opportunity to be fully involved in their care.

ACTION POINT

<u>Providers</u> should:

*   establish ways, including linkworker and advocacy schemes, of supporting women whose first language is not English to enable them to participate fully in their care.

Section 3.7

OBJECTIVE

Staff should have received training to enable them to support all women with different needs so that they can use the service to maximum advantage.

ACTION POINT

<u>Providers, statutory and professional bodies</u> should:

*   ensure that all staff have access to training which is designed to help them understand the differing needs women may have.

CHAPTER 4

Section 4.1

OBJECTIVE

Within a period of 5 years, providers should be able to demonstrate a significant shift towards a more community-oriented service.

ACTION POINT

<u>Purchasers</u> should:

*   develop strategic plans for maternity services, with guidance on future purchasing intentions showing positive moves towards woman centred and community-based care.

Section 4.2

OBJECTIVE

The views of women who use the service should be regularly monitored and services adjusted to reflect their needs.

ACTION POINT

<u>Purchasers and providers</u> should:

*   agree a monitoring system to enable them to achieve this objective.

Section 4.3

OBJECTIVE

Clinical practice should be based on sound evidence and be subject to regular clinical audit.

ACTION POINTS

<u>Purchasers</u> should:

*   agree with providers quality standards based on current evidence of effectiveness of treatment and procedures.

<u>Providers</u> should:

*   review their procedures for clinical audit.

Section 4.4

OBJECTIVE

New patterns of service should be designed to allow evaluation of both their effectiveness and their acceptability to women using the service.

ACTION POINTS

<u>Purchasers</u> should:

*   agree with providers the objectives of new approaches to providing health care and the methods for evaluating them.

Section 4.5

OBJECTIVE

The service provided must represent value for money and the cost and benefits of alternative arrangements assessed locally.

ACTION POINT

<u>Purchasers</u> should:

*   agree with providers a programme to review the use of current resources, with particular emphasis on reducing unnecessary duplication.

Annex 2

EVIDENCE TO THE EXPERT MATERNITY GROUP

The following organisations, representatives of organisations and individuals presented written evidence to the Expert Maternity Group, or attended meetings of the Group to give evidence:

Association of Anaesthetists

Association of Chartered Physiotherapists in Obstetrics and Gynaecology/Chartered Society of Physiotherapy

Association of Community Health Councils

Association for Community-Based Maternity Care

Association for Improvements in Maternity Services

Association of Radical Midwives

Mr Jack Barnes, Primary Care, Department of Health

British Association of Paediatric Surgeons

British Medical Association, Central Consultants and Specialists Committee

British Medical Association, General Medical Services Committee

British Paediatric Association

Dr Iain Chalmers, Director, Cochrane Centre

City and Hackney Health Authority Maternity Services Liaison Committee

Clinical Genetics Society

Dr H Crosskey

Mr Allan Davidson, Consultant Obstetrician and Gynaecologist, Leicester Royal Infirmary NHS Trust

Dr Janet Downer, Consultant Anaesthetist, Hillingdon Hospital, London

English National Board for Nursing, Midwifery & Health Visiting

Mr John Friend, Consultant Obstetrician and Gynaecologist, Freedom Fields Hospital, Plymouth

Mr D B Garrioch

Health Visitors Association

Independent Midwives Association

Dr Richard Jelly, Frome, Somerset

Ms Virginia Kates, consumer

Signora Bianca Lapori, Architect, Rome, Italy

Ms Nicky Leap, Independent Midwife, South East London Group Practice

Dr Philip Leech, Primary Care, Department of Health

Mr P Lewis

Dr C M Marvin

Maternity Alliance

Mr Peter Milledge, Solicitors Branch, Department of Health

Dr Barbara Morgan, Consultant Anaesthetist, Hammersmith and Queen Charlotte's Hospital, London

National Childbirth Trust

National Perinatal Epidemiology Unit

Neonatal Nurses Association

NHS Trusts Federation

Obstetric Anaesthetists Association

Patients Association

Dr Sam Richmond, Consultant Neonatologist, Sunderland DGH

Miss Anne Rider, formerly Midwife Manager, University College Hospital, London

Professor Roger Rosenblatt, Researcher, University Hospital of Wales

Royal College of Anaesthetists

Royal College of General Practitioners

Royal College of Midwives

Royal College of Obstetricians & Gynaecologists

Royal College of Physicians

Dr Anthony P Rubin, Consultant Anaesthetist, Chelsea and Westminster Hospital, London

St Bartholomew's NHS Group Maternity Services Liaison Committee

Rev A Smith

Ms Jessica Smith, Solicitors Branch, Department of Health

Ms Kate Smith, consumer

Professor Gordon Stirrat

Mr Martin Sturges, Health Authority Personnel, Department of Health

United Kingdom Central Council for Nursing, Midwifery & Health Visiting

Mr Bob Venning, Health Authority Personnel, Department of Health

Wessex Regional Health Authority GP Sub-Committee to Regional Medical Advisory Committee

Dr Andrew Wilkinson, Consultant Neonatologist, University of Oxford, John Radcliffe Hospital, Oxford

Ms Allyson Williams, Midwife Manager, University College Hospital, London

Working Mothers Association

Mr J P Wyllie

Ms Aurora Yaacov, consumer

Dr Luke Zander, Department of General Practice, St Thomas' Hospital, London

Annex 3

MATERNITY SERVICES VISITED BY THE EXPERT MATERNITY GROUP

VENUE	KEY PERSONS
Royal Bournemouth General Hospital Maternity Unit 8 January 1993	Mrs M Wheatcroft (Director of Patient Services) Mrs L Carter (Head of Midwifery Services)
Hillingdon Hospital NHS Trust Maternity Unit 4 February 1993	Miss C A Nightingale (Women's Services Manager)
Ipswich Hospital NHS Trust Maternity Unit 19 February 1993	Miss E Fern (Women's Services Manager) Mr G Thomas (Clinical Director) Mrs M Thompson (Business Manager) Clinical Midwives Senior Midwives Consumers
John Radcliffe Hospital Maternity Unit Oxford 26 March 1993	Mr M Charnock (Clinical Director, O & G) Mrs R Imhof (Acting Director, Midwifery Services) Mrs J Knowles (Clinical Practice Developments Midwife) Miss C Pepys (Senior Sister) Anaesthetist Consumers

VENUE	KEY PERSONS
Medway Health Authority Midwifery Services 22 April[1] & 18 June 1993[2]	Mrs P Rimmell[2] (Acting Head of Midwifery Services) Ms S Stewart[1] (Head of Midwifery & Gynaecological Services) Ms A Davies[1,2] (Senior Midwife) Community Midwives Consumers
Princess Alexandra Hospital Maternity Unit Harlow 1 April 1993	Miss P Wells (Assistant Director O & G) Mrs P Wilson (Consultant O & G) Midwifery Lecturers Senior Midwives Team Midwives Consumers
Princess Anne Hospital Maternity Unit Southampton 8 January 1993	Mr D J Moss (Chief Executive) Dr N Allen (Director of Public Health) Ms S Bassil Ms K Campbell (Senior Midwives) Ms J Dunne (Purchaser) Mr J Miller (Clinical Director) Mr N J Saunders Professor E J Thomas (Consultants O & G) Consumers
'Know your Midwife Scheme' Rhondda Valleys Taff Ely Health Unit Mid Glamorgan Health Authority 19 January 1993	Ms J Keats (Senior Midwife and Business Manager, Maternal and Child Services)

VENUE	KEY PERSONS
Royal London Hospital and Associated Community Services NHS Trust. Women's Services Unit 18 December 1992	Miss M Anthony (Women's Services Manager) Ms L Ahmet (Senior Midwife) Mr T Beedham Professor J G Grundzinkas Ms B Kuypers Dr L Parsons Mrs W Savage Community Midwives Consumers Health Aides (Bengali speaking)
Scunthorpe & Goole NHS Trust Scunthorpe General Hospital Maternity Unit 28 April 1993	Mrs V Outram (Director of Midwifery Services) Mrs K Chevins Mrs P Pogson Mrs K Robinson (Clinical Midwifery Managers) Mrs K Purves (Midwives Team Leader) Miss B Scott (Hospital Midwives Team Leader) Team Midwives
Sharoe Green Hospital Maternity Unit Preston 26 February 1993	Mrs C Bell (Director of Midwifery & Gynaecological Services) Mr I W Manson (Clinical Director) Consultants GPs NCT Representative Senior Midwives
South East London Group Practice Independent Midwives 5 February 1993	Ms J Demilew Ms N Leap Ms D Morris Ms R Reed Ms C Walton

VENUE

Stepping Hill Hospital
Maternity Unit
Stockport
4 December 1992

KEY PERSONS

Ms A Harrison
(Head of Midwifery Services)
Consultants
Consumers
GPs
Midwives

Annex 4

MATERNITY CARE: CHOICE, CONTINUITY AND CHANGE

CONSENSUS STATEMENT

March 1993

This statement on Britain's maternity services was drawn up by an independent panel following a consensus conference held in London on 4-5 March 1993. It was organised by the King's Fund Centre for the Department of Health.

The statement will be presented as evidence to the Expert Committee on Maternity Services set up in 1992 by Baroness Cumberlege, following the report of the Parliamentary Select Committee on Health (Winterton Report).

The panel comprised:

Niall Dickson (Chair), Chief Social Affairs Correspondent of the BBC; Akgul Baylav, Ethnic Minorities Service Manager, City and East London Family Health Services Authority; Kuldip Bharj, Senior Lecturer in Midwifery, Airedale College of Health; Sue Blennerhassett, Joint Chief Officer, Newcastle Community Health Council; Professor Richard Cooke, Professor of Paediatric Medicine, Liverpool University; Dr Lindsey Davies, Director of Public Health, Nottingham Health Authority; Catherine Griffiths, Unit General Manager, Birmingham Women's Services Unit; Rosemary Jenkins, Director of Professional Affairs, Royal College of Midwives; Dr Ann McPherson, GP, Oxford; Professor Charles Normand, Professor of Health Policy, London School of Hygiene and Tropical Medicine; Professor Gordon Stirrat, Professor of Obstetrics and Gynaecology, University of Bristol; Olivia Timbs, Editorial Director, Medicom (UK) Ltd, and mother of two children.

Invited speakers:

Margaret Anthony, Head of Women's Services, Royal London Hospital Trust; Carol Baxter, Health and Race Consultant, Manchester; Beverley Beech, Honorary Chair, Association for the Improvement of Maternity Services; Alice Coyle, Independent Midwife, London; Allan C Davidson, Consultant Obstetrician and Gynaecologist, Leicester Royal Infirmary Maternity Hospital; Karlene C Davis, Education and Midwifery Adviser, South East Thames Regional Health Authority; Ruth Evans, Director, National Consumer Council; Jo Garcia, Social Scientist, National Perinatal Epidemiology Unit, Oxford; Christine Gowdridge, Director, Maternity Alliance; John James, Chief Executive, Parkside Health Authority; Dr David Jewell, GP, Bristol, and Senior Lecturer in General Practice, Bristol University; Debra Kroll, Senior Research Officer, Community Midwifery, Bloomsbury and Islington Health Authority; Dr John McClure, Consultant Anaesthetist, Royal Infirmary, Edinburgh;

Heather Mellows, Consultant Obstetrician and Gynaecologist, Bassetlaw Hospital, Worksop, Nottinghamshire; Mary Newburn, Head of Policy Research, National Childbirth Trust; Dr John Noakes, GP, Harrow; Professor Ann Oakley, Director, Social Science Research Unit, Institute of Education, London; Professor Philip Steer, Head, Academic Department of Obstetrics and Gynaecology, Charing Cross and Westminster Medical School; Dr Jim Thornton, Senior Lecturer and Honorary Consultant Obstetrician and Gynaecologist, Leeds General Infirmary; Ann Wraight, Research Midwife, Institute of Manpower Studies.

The panel was asked to address the following questions:

1. What sort of choices are important to women and are there proper limits to women's choice as a result of clinical, organisational or financial constraints?

2. How is it possible to enhance the ability of women and their partners to make choices?

3. Women's preference is often for continuity of care and carer. Can this be described, what are the implications and how can it best be organised?

4. What are the priority actions for bringing about these changes?

A COMPREHENSIVE MATERNITY SERVICE

The overriding aims of the maternity service must be to provide the pregnant woman and her family with as safe an outcome as possible for her and her baby, to offer her choice in the type of support and care she needs and to ensure that she retains control and responsibility. Good maternity care will be built on trust between professionals and women and between the professionals themselves. It is vital that all women should have equal access to this quality of care.

It is clear, however, that there are factors beyond the scope of the maternity services, such as low incomes, poor housing and inadequate nutrition, that can have a decisive influence on a woman's experience by decreasing choice, restricting access to services and increasing risks to her and her baby. While the NHS needs to provide services which mitigate the effect of these disadvantages, there are obvious limits as to what can be done by health care alone.

1a What sort of choices are important to women?

There is considerable evidence which points to a set of universal standards that all women want from their maternity care: they have said they want a service that offers safety, that is flexible and responsive to their individual needs, which communicates effectively, and provides the information that allows informed choices. Women seek a service that is respectful, personalised and kind, gives them control and makes them feel comfortable in the sense of being at ease in the environment of childbirth and having confidence in the care that is being given.

There is also evidence that many women currently are not receiving care which meets those standards, and in particular it is clear that many are denied real choice in the types of service they are offered and in the way these are delivered. There have been many small pieces of research and observational studies in recent years which have consistently indicated that women want greater choice over matters such as where antenatal care takes place, where they have their babies, who is involved in their care and what treatment they receive. More research, especially in the form of large-scale studies, is needed to expand knowledge of the particular choices that are important to women.

It would be wrong to assume that women are a homogeneous group. What suits one will not suit another. Those who wish to hand over some decision-making to professionals should also be given that choice. Likewise, while there are women who wish to be in and out of hospital as quickly as possible, there are others who want to spend longer in hospital before returning home and others who do not want to go into hospital at all. A flexible, responsive service needs to take account of these differences.

In order to make choices we believe all women and their families need to have as full information as is available about the options open to them locally, and they need to be made aware of the benefits and risks of those options. That does present problems:

the benefits and risks of many procedures are not known and, where they are, professionals are not always good at providing objective and comprehensible explanations.

There have been significant changes in maternity care in the last ten years, not least because there has been a widespread recognition that the service needs to adapt to women's needs and choices. How universal the changes have been is difficult to gauge – there are many examples of good and innovative practices but in some places the service is not yet offering real choice. Some groups of women still face formidable barriers in securing the types and level of services that others are able to take for granted. For choice to be real there needs to be a range of services.

In some places options are limited because there simply is not the range of appropriate and skilled personnel or the care settings available. There is also evidence that sometimes women do not have full access to what is available. Often this stems from breakdowns in communication. It would be difficult to overstate the importance of providing consistent, reliable and objective information. Professional attitudes are also crucial and in some cases will need to change so that, for example, obstetric protocols are used to influence and inform good practices, and not to deny choice.

It is evident that some groups of women are offered less choice than others. Women from black and ethnic minorities, disabled women, travellers and those in poor or no housing find that choice and access which is sometimes available to others is frequently not available to them. More research is needed on the choices that are important to different groups of women, although there is no doubt that more advocates and link workers, better training and greater efforts to develop services in consultation with users will help.

Much of the discussion about choice in pregnancy has focused on those women who believe that a home birth offers them the best chance of a fulfilling experience. It is possible that more women would choose this option were it made more available, with the benefits and risks spelt out objectively alongside the benefits and risks of the alternatives. However, we believe that home confinement may have come to symbolise 'real' choice because of the more personalised service that it offers and the fact that it explicitly leaves control in the hands of the woman and her family.

1b Are there proper limits to women's choice as a result of clinical, organisational, or financial constraints?

The panel took the view that there were few justifiable constraints on women's choice and that many of those that are sometimes put forward will occur only in very exceptional circumstances.

Clinical Constraints

In particular there are few proper clinical constraints on women's freedom of choice. In rare instances choice might justifiably be denied but this is usually in response to a demand for intervention rather than a request to avoid it. For example, professionals might properly refuse to induce labour where there were no clinical grounds for so doing. There could also be situations where the woman is not in a position to make choices because her autonomy is impaired, for example if she is unconscious.

Professionals have the responsibility to give women and their partners advice based on their knowledge and experience; they do not have the right to impose their views even where they believe the mother's choice may increase the risk of harm to herself and her baby.

It is perhaps more relevant that women's choice can be constrained by the fact that professionals often do not have, and probably never will have, definitive answers on the implications of pursuing a particular course. In all this, professionals need the confidence and the communication skills to help users to make decisions in the face of uncertainty.

Organisation

Some of the current limitations on choice stem from the way services are organised but, as with clinical considerations, there are few which in practice can be justified. Many of the traditional barriers to choice, such as a lack of appropriately-skilled personnel, duplication of effort and impersonal surroundings, can be overcome and in many places the shortcomings of the past are being tackled. It should also be possible to ensure that organisational structures are geared to providing continuity of care and maximum choice.

However, even with more flexible services there will be some limits as to what can be offered. It is not possible or even desirable always to guarantee that the midwife who handles the bulk of the antenatal care will be present at the birth. This would require inappropriately long working hours. However, the organisation of the services should be such that, wherever possible, the woman knows the midwife who delivers her baby.

Resources

It is almost impossible to judge how far resources act as a constraint since there is a regrettable lack of information about the cost of existing provision or about how much would be involved in developing alternative arrangements to extend choice. There are examples where choice does appear to be restricted by a lack of resources and levels of service and the facilities available in different areas vary considerably. But there is also some evidence that changes will bring about resource savings, such as the better use of professional skills. Other changes, such as making delivery rooms more homely, could be introduced without significant extra spending.

2 How can you enhance the ability of women and their partners to make choices?

Choice is fundamental and all levels in the health service with responsibility for maternity care need to re-examine what choices are genuinely available to women and their families. Maximising choice should be a priority.

The Patient's Charter sets national standards in the provision of health services. In the case of maternity services, if choice is to be extended these need to be developed to meet the criteria of safety, responding to the needs and choices of individual women, good communication, respect and kindness. There will also need to be mechanisms to monitor the commissioning and provision of services against these national standards.

At local level, purchasers should maximise the choices available by specifying and commissioning a range of provision. They should ensure that local needs and circumstances are fully taken into account in the purchasing decisions and set quality standards within their contracts which meet the objectives already outlined. They also have a responsibility to ensure that women and their families are provided with full information on all the options for their care during and after pregnancy.

More needs to be done to involve users, and purchasers will need to develop a variety of methods to ensure that they are involved in setting priorities and in monitoring contracts. Effective Maternity Service Liaison Committees (MSLC) offer one mechanism for achieving this provided that they have adequate user representation, from bodies such as Community Health Councils, local voluntary organisations and consumer groups. They should also include, where possible, some individual mothers. MSLCs also offer the opportunity for collaboration across the professional groups.

While recognising that it is often hard to discover the preferences of different users and to make sure that less vocal interests are heard, purchasers and providers of maternity care should nevertheless make strenuous efforts to do so.

Full and unbiased information is essential if women and their partners are to make effective choices throughout pregnancy. It needs to be provided in appropriate, sensitive and understandable ways (written and oral) and should avoid overload. It should be available before, during and after pregnancy and provided in a variety of settings. There are examples of good practice, such as well-put-together information leaflets in a range of languages and imaginative use of innovative media. Information should cover all local options, women's rights, standards of care, how to gain access to appropriate services and whom women should approach if they are dissatisfied with the service. Information, in whatever form, should be open minded, non directive and where possible based on evaluated research.

The transfer of information depends on successful communication with all women. Choices for women who do not share the same language and culture as the providers must be enhanced through trained and well-resourced interpreters, advocates and link workers.

Professional training needs to stress the rights of women to make informed choices, should assist in fostering appropriate attitudes to cultural diversity and should enhance communication skills. Equal opportunities policies and practices should be reinforced by training. Team working can be enhanced through the use of common modules in the training of professionals

The quality and availability of information at the point of entry into services is crucial. General practitioners are currently the most common first point of contact and therefore have particular responsibility for making women aware of choices of services and professionals available. There is evidence that this happens only in a minority of cases, particularly in relation to some dimensions of choice, such as the place of birth.

Although it may be possible to provide some enhanced choice without additional resources, in other cases it will depend on the ability to release funds currently locked into established patterns of provision. This would require pump-priming and transitional support. Facilities may need to be developed and staff training and development carried out before new services can be introduced.

Real choices in maternity services cannot be seen in isolation from other policies. There is, for example, an important overlap with the quality and availability of family planning services to try to ensure that every pregnancy is a wanted one. The Department of Health should also liaise with other government departments to consider the impact of government policies on healthy choices and outcomes, such as the impact of benefit levels on access to healthy diets, and the impact of paid maternity leave on the feasibility of breast feeding. Paternity leave could enable men to be more involved.

3 Women's preference is often for continuity of care and carer. Can this be described, what are the implications, and how can it best be organised?

Lessons from past and recent studies point to the need for greater continuity of care and for services to be flexible enough to meet women's needs.

However, it is not clear from the evidence just how important, in itself, continuity of care is for most women. Although studies have shown that women believe it is desirable, they do not necessarily rank it as highly as, for example, having a safe delivery or receiving consistent advice. In practice though, one of the most effective ways of achieving such consistency will be to reduce the number of professional staff involved in the care of each woman and to ensure that they work together as a team. For most women the midwife will be the key professional in providing continuity and, given the preference of many women for community-based antenatal care, the aim should be to reorientate services so that midwives can follow women throughout and beyond their pregnancies. However, the provision of continuity of carer is not exclusive to any one professional group.

Description of 'continuity of care'

Continuity of care is most easily provided by one professional but in most cases it is unlikely to be achieved, and in practice there will be a spectrum of continuity. Within that lies the idea of continuity of carer which implies that the woman should have the chance to build a relationship based on trust with those looking after her throughout pregnancy, and that one of them should be available especially at crucial times such as the birth.

Implications of providing continuity of care

Movement towards greater continuity may not imply significant organisational change but it does have implications for practice. There will need to be agreed and consistent clinical policies, consistent advice to women, careful and consistent note keeping and the development of individual care plans.

Many of the current problems occur when communication breaks down between professionals, and between them and the women and their families. This can create difficulties for all women but it can be especially damaging for those with particular needs. One remedy that can at least reduce the potential for misunderstandings and confusion is to enable women to hold their own notes.

It is also vital that, if improvements are to be made in this aspect of care as in others, the standards, consistency and outcomes of the service are audited continually.

Implications for continuity of carer

Changing patterns of service to ensure continuity of carer will require more flexible working patterns as well as a fundamental change in the relationship between the care giver and the woman, with attendant emotional benefits and costs. There will also need to be changes in the relationships between professions with a greater recognition of each other's contributions. It will be important to provide support for professionals when things go wrong.

All this is certain to have significant implications for training as professional staff have to adapt to new roles and acquire a broader range of skills.

All those involved in setting up new approaches to care will have to take account of practical difficulties such as the sensitive deployment of trainees who can dilute and dislocate continuity. Reliance on part-time working and the reduction in junior doctors' hours may also have an impact on continuity of care.

Greater emphasis on midwifery as the profession most likely to provide continuity of care to the majority of women may have an impact on the systems of remuneration both for GPs and midwives.

Organisation

Continuity of care will probably best be provided by small teams of midwives with their own caseloads, working between hospital and the community and linked with primary healthcare teams.

Local services must be driven by the requirements of the woman and must be able to respond flexibly. Whether the key figure for an individual woman in the team is a midwife, GP, general obstetrician or tertiary-care specialist will depend on her particular needs and choices, although each team will have midwives able to provide the woman with maternity care irrespective of her particular additional needs.

Different models of care will be suitable for different parts of the country and we do not feel it would be appropriate to be prescriptive about the pattern of service that should be adopted. There are already primary healthcare and obstetric care teams who provide continuity of care; tertiary obstetric services have been developed in some areas but require expansion. Midwifery teams are in their infancy and greater priority should be given to their development. However, as with all other innovations, they need to be monitored and evaluated to ensure they achieve what they set out to do.

4. What are the priority actions for bringing about these changes?

In order to achieve the changes outlined in this statement, action will have to be taken at all levels in the health service. The following specific measures deserve to be highlighted:

At national level

We recommend that the Government should:

- ensure that national standards for maternity care are set;

- review the consistency of policies across government departments that impact on the health of pregnant women and babies;

- commission research into the following: women's needs and wants; the effectiveness of routine clinical procedures; the costs and effectiveness of, and satisfaction with, different models of care;

- improve routine reporting of activity (including activity of midwives) and costs of maternity services to allow audit, comparisons between and planning for service development. Such data will need to come from GPs, community and hospital services;

- develop new payment criteria for GP, hospital, midwifery and community services which will encourage more appropriate patterns of care;

provide pump-priming and transitional funds to facilitate a diverse range of care and the consequent training that will be needed to implement these changes.

We support the setting up of the Government's Maternity Services Task Force on good practice and hope that it will ensure the dissemination of high-quality information and in particular that it will see that examples of good written information for users are widely circulated so that they can be adapted for local use.

At local level

We recommend that managers should examine the whole range of maternity services and, building on existing strengths, should set goals for new development, establish a timetable for change and evaluate the outcomes.

We recommend that purchasers, including FHSAs, should:

_ undertake a fundamental review of the commissioning of maternity services against the criteria of availability of choice; local accessibility; continuity of care and diversity of need (accepting that this may result in short-term investment for long-term gain);

_ provide women and their families with a full range of unbiased information on the services available;

_ develop effective monitoring mechanisms which involve users;

_ develop mechanisms which enable pregnant women to be referred and/or transferred from one team to another (including, where reasonable, across district boundaries) depending on their changing needs or wishes.

We recommend that providers should:

_ develop and publish a service philosophy, agreed by all involved (including users themselves) placing women and their families at the centre of care;

_ develop alternative models of good practice which maximise continuity of care and foster antenatal services in the community. All such changes should take into account existing good practice in their area and evaluated research. Innovative forms of care should be encouraged but only in the context of evaluated studies;

_ collect feedback from users and involve them in the development of services. Training and support should be provided for users who participate in developing services;

- ensure consistency of advice from staff;

- maximise continuity of care for high-risk women wherever it takes place;

- ensure that boundaries between providers do not preclude the reasonable movement of women or staff in support of continuity.

Professionals

There is no place for professional rivalries which only hinder the provision of good maternity services, and it is clear that tensions do exist in some places.

We recommend that:

- professional bodies review training requirements. This would include developing the training of obstetricians in the community, and updating the training of midwives and GPs in resuscitation, examination and care of the newborn;

- training programmes should be developed for all staff to include psycho-social skills, ethics, communication (including cross-cultural), and equal opportunities. There should be shared learning involving the different professions.

There is much that is good in maternity care in this country, but it is also clear that further reform is both desirable and inevitable. The changes set out in this report represent a move towards more woman centred care in which users will be able to take part in decision making about their own care and provide feedback about their experiences to improve the service of the future.

Annex 5

NEONATAL RESUSCITATION: THE REPORT OF A BRITISH PAEDIATRIC ASSOCIATION WORKING PARTY, JUNE 1993

SUMMARY OF RECOMMENDATIONS

RECOMMENDATION 1

Midwives, neonatal nurses, general practitioners, particularly those providing obstetric care, as well as all paediatric and obstetric junior staff, should be trained in neonatal resuscitation.

Training should be given before they take up full responsibility for providing this service. They should continue to be supervised by experienced staff until their skills have been assessed as satisfactory.

Appraisal of skills and revision courses should be organised on a regular basis.

RECOMMENDATION 2

It is vital that the definition of low-risk pregnancy is agreed locally. The criteria on which the definition is based should be set out in written guidelines.

It is essential to plan that anticipated low-risk deliveries take place where sufficient trained staff and adequate resuscitation equipment are present.

It is the responsibility of the professional accepting the mother for home delivery to explain that, because of the distance from further assistance, there are some limitations to resuscitation of a newborn baby in the home.

RECOMMENDATION 3

Plans for home delivery must ensure that:

(a)   mothers know when and how to summon their birth attendant;

(b)   no delivery takes place without two trained professionals present (eg midwife and GP, or two midwives);

(c)   at least one of the professionals present is fully trained and experienced in bag and mask resuscitation of newborn babies.

RECOMMENDATION 4

Plans for delivery in a General Practitioner Maternity Unit must ensure that:

(a)   it has been agreed before the delivery who will have overall responsibility for resuscitation of the baby. Written District procedures for summoning further help should be agreed by all providers;

(b)   no delivery takes place without two members of the unit staff present in the building. One of these should be fully trained in resuscitation and be available to attend to the newborn baby if necessary.

RECOMMENDATION 5

Plans for delivery in hospital must ensure that:

(a)   within the delivery area an appropriately-trained professional is immediately available to undertake resuscitation;

(b)   high-risk deliveries should not take place where fully trained paediatric medical staff are unavailable;

(c)   there is a professional available within the hospital at all times who can maintain lung aeration by endotracheal intubation if the baby does not make a satisfactory response to mask ventilation.

RECOMMENDATION 6

The resources for the staff and equipment necessary to provide training and retraining in the techniques of neonatal resuscitation should be agreed locally.

RECOMMENDATION 7

Regular audit should be carried out of all aspects of resuscitation practice, including the availability of appropriately-trained staff and the provision of equipment.

Printed in the United Kingdom for The Stationery Office
TJ5214, C5, 8/01, 5673